EVOLUTIONARY HEALING

EVOLUTIONARY HEALING

Barbara Sarter, PhD, FNP

Associate Professor
University of Southern California

JONES AND BARTLETT PUBLISHERS
Sudbury, Massachusetts
BOSTON   TORONTO   LONDON   SINGAPORE

World Headquarters
Jones and Bartlett Publishers
40 Tall Pine Drive
Sudbury, MA 01776
978-443-5000
www.jbpub.com
info@jbpub.com

Jones and Bartlett Publishers Canada
2406 Nikanna Road
Mississauga, ON L5C 2W6
CANADA

Jones and Bartlett Publishers International
Barb House, Barb Mews
London W6 7PA
UK

Copyright © 2002 by Jones and Bartlett Publishers, Inc.

Library of Congress Cataloging-in-Publication Data

Sarter, Barbara.
    Evolutionary healing / Barbara Sarter.
       p. ; cm.
    Includes bibliographical references and index.
     ISBN 0-7637-1808-4
     1. Health—Philosophy. 2. Healing—Philosophy. 3.
Medicine—Philosophy. 4. Consciousness. 5. Mind and
body—Health aspects.
    [DNLM: 1. Mind-Body Relations (Metaphysics). 2. Religious
Philosophies. WB 880 S249e 2002] I. Title.
    R723 .S226 2002
    610'.1--dc21   2002029709

Production Credits
Acquisitions Editor: Penny M. Glynn
Associate Editor: Christine Tridente
Production Editor: Anne Spencer
Editorial Assistant: Thomas Prindle
Manufacturing Buyer: Amy Duddridge
Cover Design: Anne Spencer
Design and Composition: Carlisle Communications, Ltd.
Printing and Binding: Malloy Lithographing

Printed in the United States of America
05 04 03 02 01   10 9 8 7 6 5 4 3 2 1

DEDICATION

To all those who suffer.

INTRODUCTION

I am writing this book after 25 years of caring for people from all walks of life and innumerable cultures. It is a reflection of my personal quest to come to terms with the meaning of human suffering. In nursing school I began asking, "Why do people suffer so much? Why is there so much illness and tragedy in our world?" I knew from deep within that there was something very special shining in the faces of the sick and dying. They looked purified and real. They possessed a dignity that only suffering brings. I was drawn to their bedsides. I wanted to learn from them.

As I tested my wings as a nurse, my search intensified. I began to study the spiritual views of the great sages and saints from all spiritual and philosophical traditions. After witnessing the complexities of mental illness as a psychiatric nurse, I moved into intensive care, then into oncology nursing, where my search became truly urgent. Then I saw young people, even children, going through enormous suffering and dying after heroic struggles. After being with a patient, I often would dash into the bathroom at Memorial Sloan-Kettering Cancer Center and burst into tears. My heart ached and my soul agonized over the plight of those I cared for. As I went through graduate school and completed my doctorate, my scholarly research focused on these same issues from a formal, philosophical point of view.

Gradually, insight began to dawn. I came to understand that life is a process of spiritual growth, of the growth of consciousness. In this process, suffering and death often are of more value than are happiness and health. I needed to take a very large view, beyond the time frame of a single life. The inner self is always undergoing refinement, life after life, until it reaches perfection and no longer needs the lessons of earth. The hard knocks of illness and suffering have a purpose to serve. They are our teachers. They help us move on. They help deepen and expand our awareness. This is the beauty I saw in the faces of those who were suffering. It was the purification of their souls.

This book is the culmination of my life as a nurse, scholar, and seeker. It integrates ancient and modern philosophies of life—commonly known as the *perennial philosophy*—with modern scientific discovery. I apply these philosophies to the process of healing and describe what I have come to call *evolutionary healing*. Evolutionary healing is the evolution of one's consciousness through health and disease.

Throughout this book, I refer to levels or spheres of existence. This needs some explanation. The *great chain of being* was the unifying paradigm of medieval European thought. This chain was more like a ladder, with the lowest rung holding human beings and the highest rung, God. Angels and other celestial beings were in between. There was no movement from one rung to another.

In the scientific era, we lost sight of these otherworldly phenomena and described a chain of biological evolution, from amoebas to humans. The chain became a branching tree. Darwin redefined history by demonstrating that there is a gradual development, or unfolding, of the later and more complex forms from the earlier, simpler forms. I am extending this tree of evolution from the creation of our universe to the divine, the source and the culmination of the entire process. I maintain that there is evolutionary movement from inanimate to animate to human to divine. These levels of existence are distinct spheres, each having its own laws and principles, each building on the previous one. But they are all made of the same stuff: conscious energy. In the time frame of the universe, the inanimate sphere is the oldest, and the human the youngest. The divine is beyond time and space; it is eternal.

I would like to acknowledge my primary sources. The school of thought I call *evolutionary idealism* or *evolutionary spiritualism* has been most helpful in shedding light on the meaning of human suffering. Three 20th-century philosophers from this tradition had a major influence on my work: Aurobindo Ghosh[1], Swami Ramananda[2,3,4], and Pierre Teilhard de Chardin[5,6,7]. Aurobindo and Ramananda were philosophers and spiritual masters from India. Both were born into the Hindu tradition but transcended the confines of religious dogma to expound synthetic, comprehensive views of cosmic and human evolution. Teilhard was a Jesuit priest and distinguished paleontologist, and from this background he developed an evolutionary view similar to that of Aurobindo and Ramananda. To these three I owe the inspiration for the basic philosophy of this book. Behind these three philosophers is a long tradition of evolutionary philosophers whose ideas provided food for thought. The spiritual successor to Ramananda, Prince Kumar, has been my constant inspiration and makes the ideas of evolutionary spiritualism directly applicable to daily life.

The scientific work of Stuart Kauffman[8,9], Rupert Sheldrake[10,11,12], Fritjof Capra[13,14], and Ilya Prigogine[15] was also crucial to this synthesis. The work of biologist Michael Denton[16] and physicist Paul Davies[17] was particularly helpful, as well. Michael Murphy's[18] comprehensive discussion of the evidence for human evolutionary transformation was another valuable source of data.

Finally, I must acknowledge the inspiration provided by my nursing mentor, Dr. Martha Rogers[19-22]. Her pioneering work in developing the science of unitary human beings first made me realize that a philosophy of health requires a comprehensive view of the universe and of humanity's place in it. I am proud to be following in her footsteps.

CONTENTS

CHAPTER 1

THE EVOLVING UNIVERSE

We are the universe. The universe is in us, and we are in the universe. So, in order to understand ourselves, we must understand the larger reality. The laws of health and illness reflect the laws of order and disorder in the universe. In this chapter, we examine some fundamental questions about the universe. Of what is the universe made? What principles guide the constant change we see everywhere? Our discussion draws upon many sources of knowledge including, but not limited to, scientific understanding.

Science is limited by the capacity of our senses and instruments and by the limits of the reasoning mind. Reason is certainly a necessary, but not sufficient, tool for comprehending the universe. Pure reason is rare; it is subject to the temperament, desires, and ego of the thinker. Philosophers from the upanishadic rishis to Socrates to Wittgenstein have shown us that, through logic, we eventually confront a reality beyond the reach of reason and language. This reality seems to underlie and also transcend the visible universe. At this point we must abandon logic. We must find other paths to a deeper knowledge of our world.

THE EVOLUTION OF CONSCIOUS ENERGY

The physical world consists of energy in various forms. Energy is the capacity to create change. Wherever there is change, or the potential for change, there is energy. By this definition, energy is not only a physical phenomenon. It is also the foundation of the emotional, mental, social, and spiritual spheres. Our stance is that there is a single energy underlying the entire world of becoming, though it possesses vastly different properties at various levels of manifestation. Being of the same fundamental nature, all spheres of existence can, and do, interact freely with each other.

Since the 1970s, researchers from diverse disciplines have abandoned the notion that energy is a mechanical, passive force. Quite the contrary, it appears that energy is self-organizing[8, 9, 15], has an innate tendency toward order[9, 14, 16, 17, 23], and evolves spontaneously into increasingly complex forms[8, 9, 10, 14, 15, 19–22]. Though there is a high degree of unpredictability in the way energy self-organizes, energy can create order out of apparent chaos[25].

1

This intriguing discovery causes us to ponder further on the nature of energy. Is there a mental component of energy? How does it know what form to take, what makes it want to organize itself, and why does it prefer certain patterns? Our answers to these questions form the central thesis of this book. Energy is conscious. The universe is made of conscious energy.

Consciousness is awareness. Perception is the essential activity of awareness. An entity is aware when it perceives. How do we know that perception has occurred? We know it has occurred when there are reactions and responses. And we find reactions, complex reactions, and interactions at every level of the universe. Perception and awareness—hence, consciousness—are present in all forms of energy.

In its more developed forms, we find three clearly distinguishable aspects of consciousness: knowing, willing, and feeling. Knowing is taking in the environment. Willing is acting upon the environment. Feeling is acting upon oneself, or self-modification. We see vague stirrings of knowing and willing in the rudimentary signals and interactions among quantum particles. Radioactivity gives us a glimpse of self-modification, or feeling. An element transforms itself while emitting radioactive energy.

From these elementary particles we can trace the development of knowing-willing-feeling through chemical bonding, the formation of cells, the intelligent adaptation of plants, the complex physiological integration of animals, and the sophisticated social behavior and spiritual exploration of humans. We see an unbroken chain of consciousness extending from the origin of the universe to humankind and beyond.

Energy evolves. Evolution originally was a biological theory, but it has now been expanded to apply to all levels of the universe. In every sphere, change shows definite patterns and tendencies. Evolution implies the unfolding of a latent potential. In the history of our universe we see increasing complexity of form, starting from the big bang, to the formation of heavier atoms, to the formation of primitive cells by the combination of more and more complex molecules. From here on the story is well known. Biological evolution demonstrates a strong tendency toward increasing complexity of form and function. Underlying this increasing complexity is an increase in consciousness.

Our position is that the evolution of consciousness is the primary event of the entire process. Here we find a fundamental difference between the materialist and idealist philosophers. The materialist insists that the evolution of consciousness is a by-product of the evolution of form. The idealist maintains that the evolution of form is the vehicle for the evolution of consciousness. We see in the human sphere that consciousness has evolved to such a degree that it has the capacity to regulate the evolutionary process that produced it. Conscious values dominate human life. We are now in a position to manipulate genes, one of the main vehicles of evolution.

The idealist view of the situation explains more of the facts and supports our deepest intuitions about the nature of reality. It is a view expressed in every age by sages, philosophers, and mystics. This view of evolution bestows on existence a meaning and purpose. And, from every age, we have shining examples of the possibility of further evolution beyond our ordinary human consciousness.

There really is very little debate over the fact that, as evolution proceeds, consciousness is increasing in breadth and depth. The issue is whether this is purely by chance or whether it is part of some grand design in the universe. Let us take a closer look at the materialist hypothesis that chance events combined with natural selection have been the mechanisms of evolution on the earth. First, we must accept that random events resulted in the formation of living cells. Next, we must believe that aimless mutations in our ancestors' genetic structures, starting from the amoebas, led ultimately to the formation of a complex human organism with a nervous system. The tenets of materialism are contrary to our common sense and to our deepest intuitions about the value of human life and the life of all beings.

New insights and discoveries from the last few decades have shaken the edifice of scientific materialism—even among its staunch supporters. We have a new generation of scientists saying that self-organization, not randomness, is the mechanism of evolutionary change[8, 9, 15, 25]. Biologists have shown that mutations occur specifically in response to certain needs of the organism, rather than just randomly. The paradox of chaos theory is that, in every arena, there is order and pattern, even in apparently random processes.

Kauffman[8, 9] has shown us that the evolution of complex systems actually is more likely to occur as they become chaotic. When a system becomes disorganized, it is more likely to reorganize into a higher degree of complexity than if it remains in its earlier state. Even subatomic systems appear to behave this way. Systems naturally move into more complex patterns. The result of this increased complexity is an increase in the informational capacity of the system. It can know more, experience deeper feeling, and act more effectively upon its environment. An evolving system becomes more conscious.

Physicist David Bohm[23, 24] called the order underlying the world of apparently random events the *implicate order*. The implicate order is a world of wholeness and meaning, where everything is interconnected. Seemingly lawless or random events reveal their inner logic or meaning in the implicate order. Similarly, Sheldrake[10, 11] maintains that invisible *morphic fields* organize and regulate not only the orderly development of individual organisms but also the evolution of the millions of species on the earth. Kauffman, Bohm, and Sheldrake also imply that consciousness is present in the physical universe.

Complexity and consciousness, then, increase as evolution proceeds. We noted that as evolution proceeds consciousness becomes the dominant factor in life. It emerges as the strongest influence in the arena of human life. The arts and philosophy, values, and ideals inspire and shape our world.

Spiritual experience, especially near-death experience, affirms that consciousness is present even after the body is dead. The research of Melvin Morse[26] and Raymond Moody[27] carefully documents thousands of cases of near-death experiences. Their interviews with children and adults who have had these experiences reveal a remarkable consistency in the insights gained. These include the understanding that an individual's life on earth is just one phase of existence; consciousness does continue after death.

It is not so difficult then to conclude that the evolution of consciousness is the driving force behind the evolution of our universe. Consciousness is unfolding; it is pressing forth to express itself ever more fully. This will be our primary assumption as we explore the relationship between healing and evolution.

When we see the violence and inhumanity of modern civilization, it appears that human consciousness is on a path of decline rather than of advancement. Many philosophers and historians have reflected on the paradox that in this century we have achieved tremendous potential not only for good, but also for harm. Jean Gebser[28], influenced by Aurobindo[1], identified five stages of human evolution: archaic, magical, mythical, mental, and integral. Each stage marks a structural transformation in human consciousness. Unrest, violence, and ignorance characterize the transitions between stages. They are transitions on the edge of chaos. But, as discussed previously, chaotic transitions are fertile ground for the emergence of increasing complexity and consciousness. They are the storms of adolescence before the maturity of adulthood is reached.

Gebser[28] describes the integral stage of human evolution as one of global awareness. He believes that we are just entering this stage. Aurobindo[1] calls this stage *supramental* and Ramananda[2] calls it *wisdom*. All agree that it is characterized by transcendence of the individual ego, a universal sympathy, and identification with the larger universe.

In the evolutionary paradigm, each new level of development subsumes all the earlier levels. The earlier structures, patterns, and operations are integrated into the new stage. Thus, it is important that we examine the structure and characteristics of each stage of evolution that preceded the human stage, for herein we will find important insights into our own nature, including insights into the laws of health and illness.

ELEMENTAL CONSCIOUSNESS

Subatomic and atomic particles, atoms, minerals, chemicals and compounds, and complex molecules make up the elemental world. The consciousness of the elements is rudimentary. Their reactions and interactions are largely automatic, in accordance with the laws of physics and chemistry. Even the self-organization of the elements is in accordance with physical laws.

But our understanding of physical laws is changing. The new physics offers us a vision of a dynamic universe, rather than the mechanical universe of classical physics. Capra[13] was the first to articulate this new vision: "In this world, classical concepts like 'elementary particles', 'material substance', or 'isolated object', have lost their meaning; the whole universe appears as a dynamic web of inseparable energy patterns" (pp. 83, 85).

The physical universe is made of electromagnetic energy fields. Electromagnetic fields have no real boundaries. Their energy exists in a pattern called a *probability distribution*. This means that there are different degrees of probability that the energy of a given field will be concentrated in certain areas. But, theoretically, a field's energy extends infinitely—as far as the boundaries of the universe. The current view is that the universe's boundary is expanding constantly. Some physicists believe that this expansion will continue forever, whereas others maintain that the universe goes through repeating cycles of expansion and contraction.

The fields making up our universe, having infinite boundaries, obviously are interpenetrating. In fact, we can no longer think of distinct entities such as atoms or even particles as composing the universe. Electromagnetic fields are better described as processes in constant interaction with each other, forming new fields with different patterns of energy.

It is helpful to think of the world as consisting of vibrations. Physics has shown us that electromagnetic fields have wave-like properties as well as particle-like properties. They behave as particles when measured by scientific instruments. But their patterns of distribution have the mathematical form of waves. Waves undulate, or vibrate. The vibrations of various energy fields vary only in their frequency. Elemental energy vibrates at a slower rate than do the energies that evolved later. This is why we can see it either with the naked eye or with our scientific instruments.

In this universe of energy fields with interpenetrating infinite boundaries, nonlocal interactions among fields are possible. *Nonlocal interaction* means action at a distance. Classical physics maintains that only objects in proximity to each other can influence each other. But an object is actually an energy field without real boundaries. It can affect all the other energy fields in the universe because it is intertwined with all others. Evidence is mounting that this is indeed the case.[29]

Space and time were separate realities in the world of classical physics. In the new physics, they lose their independent status. Einstein demonstrated the relativity of space and time. Capra[13] explains that "space is curved to different degrees and time flows at different rates in different parts of the universe" (p. 187). We are accustomed to measuring and manipulating the physical world using concepts of three-dimensional space and linear time. On a practical level, in everyday life, this works quite well. But if we move into the infinitesimally small world of quantum particles or into the vast universe thousands of light-years in breadth, we find that ordinary space and time become irrelevant. We also find that, as we move from the physical world into the other levels of existence like mind or spirit, space and time lose their relevance.

Another challenge to our usual way of thinking comes from new insights into the nature of subatomic particles. Normally, we believe that two opposite qualities cannot exist at the same time in the same event or object. But, at the subatomic level, Capra[13] explains, "particles are both destructible and indestructible. . . . Matter is both continuous and discontinuous, and force and matter are but different aspects of the same phenomenon" (p. 152). We saw earlier that energy also exists as both particles and waves. Paradox, then, seems to be a fundamental quality of our world. This is difficult for the reasoning mind to grasp.

The uncertainty principle also bears mention in this overview of elemental consciousness. Briefly, this is the finding, in subatomic physics, that one can never know with certainty both the position and the momentum of a particle. If we measure the position precisely, the momentum will be unmeasurable, and vice versa. Scientists used to think that they could measure events in the physical world precisely and accurately. But the key insight of the uncertainty principle is that the very act of measurement influences the properties of the subject. The observer can never be detached, he or she is instead always a participant in the process.

The above insights from the new physics tell us that the elemental world is by no means inanimate. It is a world full of movement, of self-organized spontaneous activity, of definite tendencies to react and interact in distinctive patterns. The elements of our visible world have unique properties, reacting in certain ways to different elements. Carbon, for example, is a highly reactive element that combines with many others, whereas boron is very inert, showing very little bonding capacity. Ramananda[2] comments, "This capacity to react in a distinctive manner shows that there must be some registration of the stimulus, or else how could a definite pattern of behavior be possible? This indicates the presence of consciousness in atoms" (p. 49). Truly, our universe is alive!

Of course, all three aspects of consciousness are at a primitive stage in the elemental world. Here, cognition is limited to perception. No intelligent activity is possible, as far as we know. Will, or conation, is minimal, although some choice is allowed in the presence of randomness. Affection or self-modification is seen in the self-organizing tendencies of physical systems. The essential qualities of consciousness are present. The potential is mostly undeveloped, but the seed is most definitely present.

ORGANIC CONSCIOUSNESS

Life is a profoundly more active and effective consciousness than is its elemental predecessor. Organic consciousness organizes and orchestrates the myriad interactions of billions of elements in order to create a functioning organism. Even the most jaded biologist is astounded at its ingenious adaptability. It goes to great lengths in order to maintain the integrity of an organism.

Organic consciousness engages in purposeful activity. Its primary goal is self-preservation. The instinct to reproduce is a broader extension of this goal. It also seeks more extensive and varying interaction with the environment and more effective resistance to hostile forces. This requires greater complexity and diversity of the organism. Thus, we have the fascinating story of biological evolution.

Organic consciousness displays great intelligence and comprehension of the environment. Special sense organs evolve to increase this cognitive aspect of consciousness. Living organisms have a tenacious will to live. All other activities are subservient to this will. Affection is also clearly present. Organisms seek stimuli that support life and avoid those that do not. A natural zest for pleasure develops. To have more pleasure, organic energy seeks ever more variety and intensity in its interactions. Thus, we find the three aspects of consciousness clearly active at the organic level.

The evolution of organic consciousness shows other tendencies besides increasing complexity of structure and function. Differentiation and specialization accompany greater complexity. Organs and systems develop. The nervous system becomes more centralized with evolution. This provides the foundation for higher manifestations of consciousness. Environmental activity also becomes more complex. The organism engages in more extensive and intensive interaction with its physical surroundings and with other organisms.

Some biologists, most notably Stephen Jay Gould[30], maintain that the trend of increasing complexity is a myth. They see only a trend toward diversity. Gould is adamant that there is no direction or purpose in evolution. But can diversity increase without an increase in complexity? It can only do so in a very limited manner. The reality of increasing complexity in evolution is undeniable. So, in fact, this distinction between diversity and complexity has little bearing on the ultimate outcome, which is the evolution of consciousness through the evolution of complexity.

Another fascinating characteristic of higher organisms is their spontaneous embryonic development from a single cell into a highly differentiated, complex organism. Equally intriguing is the way that members of a species are able to learn and share new patterns of behavior even when the former are physically very distant from each other. The 100th monkey phenomenon discussed by Sheldrake[10] is a well-known example of this learning at a distance.

Briefly, a monkey on one island starts to use a stick to collect ants from anthills. He inserts a stick into an anthole and the ants crawl up the stick; the monkey then raises the stick to his mouth and licks off the ants. The other monkeys on the island observe this successful and efficient way of collecting dinner and quickly adopt the same practice. This is understandable. But how does one explain the fact that within a short time monkeys on other islands, with no geographic link to the original island, begin to adopt the same behavior when it has never been a part of their repertoire in the past?

Sheldrake[10] hypothesizes that nonmaterial morphogenetic fields are responsible for this phenomenon of distant communication and coordinated behavior among members of a species. He has accumulated substantial evidence to support this hypothesis. Sheldrake maintains that morphogenetic fields transmit species-specific information that guides both individual and group behavior. Sheldrake describes a group consciousness unique to each species, a consciousness that evolves as experience accumulates and that governs the individual consciousness of its members.

Efforts by materialists to explain all the complex operations of life in terms of physical and chemical processes fail. Although these explanations become more and more elaborate, they never fully explain why the myriad chemical and electromagnetic processes in living organisms are so clearly goal oriented. We must admit that there is purposive consciousness present in organic energy. It is responsible for the evolutionary leap from the elements to life.

Denton[16], a contemporary molecular biologist, explains how the physical properties of the universe are precisely designed to support the emergence of carbon-based molecular structures on earth. The physical characteristics of the primitive earth were exactly what were needed to form DNA, the basis of living cells. Climatic and geologic conditions were then ideal for the evolution of more and more complex organisms. Denton concludes that the origin of life was built into the laws of nature from the beginning; it was not a random occurrence. Further, the universe has been set up from the beginning to create and support human life. It could not have arisen without a very precise, specific combination of elements and conditions. Scientists like Denton and many others are helping us realize with increasing humility that the universe is permeated with an intelligent, purposive consciousness.

Human Consciousness

It is truly astounding that many scientists are still attempting to reduce human consciousness to electrical and chemical brain processes. Fantastic theories are proposed to explain how neural connections and electrochemical processes cause the endlessly subtle depths of human thought and emotion. Scientists at many different centers throughout the world are trying to make computers that can perform the way our minds do. Yet such efforts are far from accomplishing their goal, simply because it is an impossible goal.

Intuitively, the ordinary person understands this. It is the scientific ego that destroys common sense. Anyone who looks within with a clear eye will feel the inner self that is the subject of all experience, the one that is peering out behind the sense organs and the brain. Consciousness is a principle in its own right. It is the foundation of all that exists. Consciousness makes the brain do what it does. Cognitive scientists have it backwards. The brain is a vehicle of expression for mind, which is an independent entity, a principle of evolving, conscious energy.

Self-awareness characterizes human consciousness. It is not apparent in the organic realm. Self-awareness leads to all that we know as humans. To it we owe the presence of human culture and civilization. It is generally believed that humans are the only animals who have an awareness of death. This is also due to our self-awareness.

With the dawn of self-awareness, the search for pleasure also assumes a new status. It becomes desire. Under the influence of mind, humans seek ever more intense and extensive pleasures. Desire is the dominant factor in human life. It is responsible for all behaviors that we call human. From the arts and entertainment, to science and philosophy, to war and politics, desire is the motivating force. It leads to all the effort that an individual makes to improve the conditions of life. It motivates the healing arts. Its influence is pervasive. It is a force to be reckoned with. Animal instincts are geared toward the preservation of life. Human desires, however, often become destructive of life. This is the irony of human existence. Our tastes become perverted. Our behavior becomes self-defeating.

Emotion and reason are two aspects of mental consciousness. The emotional mind has the ability to form concepts from sense perceptions. This gives it immense power over the latter, for concepts in turn can influence perceptions. The emotional mind lights up and fills in raw sensory data. It is also capable of imagination, of combining concepts in infinitely creative ways. It is responsible for great achievements in science, art, and literature. As humankind evolves, emotions gradually replace instincts and become the primary determinants of behavior. Desires form the axis around which emotions revolve.

Intensity of feeling increases and emotions deepen as a culture or individual evolves. Emotions replace physical sensations as the primary sources of pleasure and pain. Noble ideals and values are formed. The emotional mind evolves from negative, destructive emotions to positive, constructive emotions. Hatred, anger, jealousy, and fear harm the physical organism, uproot reason, and cause immense suffering in the individual and the society. Love, sympathy, and kindness gradually replace the negative emotions as the individual grows—though for a long time the two sides are in conflict and create an inner turmoil.

Emotions make the human personality distinctively individual. Among animals we find relatively little variation in personality, though differences do exist within the higher species. But emotions deepen and become so much more varied in human beings that we can truly say that each person is unique. Gradually, as we evolved from our prehuman ancestors, a set of individuals with a herd mentality was replaced by individuals who share a common culture but are capable of feeling and thinking on their own. We often find, however, that mass culture drowns individuality. It is often an insult to evolution.

Reasoning mind appears in the evolutionary process after emotional mind and is capable of restraining the latter. Reason can move beyond concept formation to the development of abstract ideas and ideals having no direct referent to sensory perception. Its thought processes are an association of concepts and ideas. Reason can discriminate among ideas, induce and deduce new ideas, and build enduring ideals. It is the foundation of science and philosophy.

Aurobindo[1] explains that reason "is a consciousness which measures, limits, cuts out forms of things from the indivisible whole and contains them as if they were a separate integer" (p. 162). Similarly, Ramananda[2] points out that reason is capable only of a three-dimensional understanding. It is able only to comprehend facts that occur in time and space. It can know opposites only as separate, never allowing that they may exist simultaneously.

Reason fortifies will. A person of strong mind can choose to behave in accordance with what he or she considers to be good. Reason also intensifies the ego. A sense of superiority and separation from others develops. This allows latent desires to be activated, and an inner struggle ensues. Others react, and ultimately a most intense inner suffering takes place.

As the person evolves and experiences the suffering born of egoism and endless desires, a higher degree of self-awareness is born. He or she begins to realize the limitations of reason and of a life based on selfish egoism. The struggle between desires and negative emotions on the one hand and reasoned self-restraint on the other creates chaos within and without. The ground is being prepared for the next step in the evolution of consciousness.

Mental vibrations are subtler than, and can regulate, to some degree, organic and emotional vibrations. But the mind cannot fulfill or integrate the person. That task is reserved for the next evolutionary stage. Ramananda[2] points out that an excess of reason "makes life dry and dull, almost inhuman. It kills emotions and starves life" (p. 96). It is self-limiting and arrogant to assume that reason is the highest possible form of knowing. A life dominated by reason leads to the inner and outer chaos that marks our current civilization. Industrialized countries have the highest suicide rates on record. Millions of people feel trapped and alienated, believing there is no way out of their isolation. They live in societies without heart, without spirit. Reason is not the pinnacle of human capability.

The development of a higher consciousness is the key to resolving the terrible predicaments of modern life. Without this possibility, we would be justified in sinking into despair. But numerous persons from all times and cultures have experienced a consciousness free of the contradictions and limitations of the mind. We will call it *superhuman consciousness*, because it is so different from ordinary human consciousness. It is characterized first by wisdom and then by love.

SUPERHUMAN CONSCIOUSNESS

Wisdom resolves the contradictions and chaos that accompany a life that is torn between emotion and reason. It is rooted in a unified vision of things, a deeper understanding and identification with one's environment, a state in which diversity and dichotomies are absorbed. Wisdom knows things directly. It need not deduce or induce. It comprehends things as a whole, rather than analyzing their parts separately. Intuition rather than analysis is its way of knowing. It can penetrate the barriers of time and space.

Wisdom also apprehends an unmanifest reality—one that is beyond the reaches of the senses. The visible universe is characterized by constant change. We can say that it is a realm of *becoming*. But we can only know change in relation to something unchanging. For example, we only know motion if there is something stationary with which to compare it. There must be a changeless background or substrate supporting this universe. This we can call *being*. Wisdom apprehends this invisible, changeless ground of existence. It can grasp both being and becoming without seeing them as mutually contradictory.

The ego begins to fade with the onset of wisdom. There is no sense of doing anything or being anything. Personal desires lose their grip. The person of wisdom desires only the well-being of all.

As desire dwindles, inner chaos subsides. There is an unshakable peace. Negative emotions fade, and the emotional mind loses its hold on the personality. An inner stability is present in the midst of all the pleasures and pains of life. Hope and anxiety cease. A universal sympathetic awareness is born. The vibrations of wisdom refine and transform all the other energies that came before it.

Many thoughtful people in contemporary society recognize that a consciousness higher than mind is necessary to solve the problems of our world. Though they may call this form of consciousness by different names, they all recognize the same possibility. Ancient spiritual philosophies of the East are attracting Western spiritual seekers in increasing numbers. This trend began in America with Thoreau and Emerson, but it is now part of our common culture. The deep ecology movement is urging a consciousness rooted in the unity of all beings, living and nonliving. The human ego that looks upon itself as controller of the environment has no place in this view.

Our most brilliant scientists have also seen through the limits of the human mind. Einstein[31] believed in a reality that the mind could not reach. He felt that this unmanifest reality was the source of order in nature. Eddington[32], Schrodinger[33], and Jeans[34]—all on the cutting edge of physics early in the 20th century—also shared similar reflections. It seems that most of the brilliant minds of our century have recognized that reason has its limits.

The establishment of wisdom consciousness prepares the person for love, the pinnacle of the evolutionary process. Love is the highest consciousness we know. This love is not the human emotion we commonly call *love*. Human love is a source of great joy, but it can also lead to intense suffering. Suffering is not possible when love is fully established. Love makes no demands, for it is self-fulfilled and blissful. It sees all and the self as part of one supreme consciousness. The sense of self and not self vanishes. Love is a consciousness few have attained in our collective human history, but there are well-known examples of mystics, saints, and realized beings who demonstrate its definite possibility.

Initially, the experience of love comes and goes, but when fully established it assumes a hold on the entire being and permeates every atom of the person. Its vibrations are so powerful that a total transformation must take place. Jesus Christ is certainly the most famous example of this transformation in the West. Buddha's enlightenment is another inspiring example.

From the point of view of evolutionary spiritualism, we are all on the path toward this epiphany. No doubt it is a painstaking process. We need to understand how the evolutionary change that leads ultimately to love actually happens, for it seems difficult, if not impossible, to accomplish in a single lifetime.

MECHANISMS OF EVOLUTION

Reincarnation

When we look around us and see the flaws and downright evil of ordinary human life, it is difficult to believe that love is our destiny. We see little evidence to support this thesis. This confusion is due in part to the absence of the idea of reincarnation from our cultural belief system. Without reincarnation, life makes little sense. We are unable to explain why some people are so good or happy or successful and why others are not. Why do some very good people suffer greatly, and some very bad people enjoy life's best rewards?

We resort to gene theory to explain our differences, but we are unable to actually demonstrate how DNA guides every detail of our behavior. If we look to upbringing and sociocultural factors, the same problems exist. Even identical twins have different personalities and fates. Reincarnation explains the variety of human behavior and circumstances better than any other concept does. We also have convincing evidence of its reality.

Reincarnation requires belief in the soul, the part of the person that we intuitively experience as our inner self. The soul is simply the unit of conscious energy. Experience accumulates in the soul, whether it be the group soul of animal species or the individuated human soul. The soul is eternal, never born and never dying. Like energy, consciousness is neither created nor destroyed. Conscious energy, then, neither is born nor dies. But the soul does evolve, and it evolves on earth through the bodies it successively takes on. This successive incarnation of the soul is called *reincarnation*.

The soul requires a variety of experience in order to grow. It requires a vast accumulation of physical, emotional, and mental experiences before it can evolve into wisdom and love. The evolution of consciousness is the evolution of the soul. Physical experience, requiring great force in order to evoke a reaction, is dynamic and far-reaching. For example, it makes no evolutionary sense for a human to incarnate as an animal. The further development of human consciousness would not be possible in an animal brain. Reincarnation is an evolutionary, educative, and cumulative process.

Researchers from around the world have provided extensive evidence for reincarnation. The evidence lies in memories of past lives. Dr. Ian Stevenson[35] at the University of Virginia is a leading researcher in this field. He has compiled several volumes of carefully validated reports of past lives. Stevenson has developed strict criteria for validating memories of past lives.

Karma

This brings us to the other missing link in our explanation of human diversity, the concept of karma. In its broadest sense, *karma* simply means action. Karma is responsible for the creation and evolution of the universe. It causes the interplay between being and becoming. Beginning with the elemental stage of evolution, it is expressed in the form of action and reaction. The complex interactions between the unit of conscious energy and its environment, the forces and laws of nature, express karma at the elemental and organic level.

Karma has a twofold effect on the individual. There is a direct reaction on the agent and an indirect reaction from the environment. The inner modification that leads to an action leaves a direct impression on the individual and may have extensive effects. For example, anger causes an act of violence directed toward the environment, but it also has an impact on the person who is angry. Repeated actions create deeply ingrained habits.

An action also comes back indirectly to the individual in the form of a response from the environment. There is another inner adjustment. By action, or karma, then, we are remolding ourselves constantly. This process goes on from the elemental to the human levels. It is the driving force behind evolution. Action and reaction speed up as evolution proceeds. The more intense the activity, the faster the evolution. Thus, we see that the pace of evolution has increased through the millennia.

Often, karma is interpreted as predestination, the idea that we have no freedom and no responsibility in our action. The contrary is true. At the human level, karma becomes a vehicle for conscious choice, creativity, and rapid self-improvement. Will becomes strong. A person has the capacity to make mistakes, suffer, learn from the mistakes, and change actions. This brings the possibility of a rapid evolution of consciousness.

Karmic reactions are very complex in humans because of the multiple layers of consciousness. A single action has repercussions in all the layers. This is a critical concept for our later discussion of health and healing. Our emotions and thoughts affect our physical organism and vice versa.

Even a simple action like eating is full of complex associations. It evokes the organic response of digestion. Like or dislike of the food is its mental response. Dislike in turn diminishes digestion and may cause stomach pains. The cook may be blamed. Indirectly, a vast network of people contribute to the meal that sits on the table—from the farmer, to the steelworker who made the farm equipment, to the trucker, and so on. Thus, an incredibly elaborate web of action and reaction is built around each human activity. Truly, we are all connected.

Now we need to bring reincarnation into the picture as well. Karmic responses and connections do not die with the physical body of a person. They remain with the evolving unit of conscious energy and explain, to a great extent, the diversity of experience and circumstance we see, especially at the human level. It is important also to understand that karmic reactions are not blind and mechanical. They operate toward a single goal: the evolution of consciousness. There is an intelligence and purpose governing the entire process. However, because the process extends beyond the boundaries of a single life, we cannot always appreciate it. As our own consciousness evolves, we begin to intuit these things directly.

Ramananda[2] provides an analysis of how karma actually operates. Reactions occur immediately only at the physical level. At the organic level—and even more so at the emotional and mental levels—reactions occur only under appropriate conditions and to the extent that they are needed for the evolution of the individual. A karmic reaction may wait several lifetimes before it finds the right opportunity to express itself. Karmic reactions bring the soul into earthly existence again and again, awakening and deepening consciousness with every return. Eventually these reactions and ties begin to lessen, as action is done not from the motivation of desire and ego but from a sense of duty or worship. Wisdom consciousness dawns. Ramananda[3] says simply, "Wisdom is the state of karmaless activity" (p. 160). Without the ties of karma, the soul may be ready to graduate from the school of human life.

THE LAWS OF EVOLUTION

Action and reaction between a unit of evolving conscious energy and its environment are the primary means and indicators of evolutionary progress. The effectiveness of action and intensity of interaction increase as complexity and consciousness evolve. Several laws govern the evolutionary development of complexity and consciousness. They are derived from the principles of biological evolution, but they are applicable to a much wider range of phenomena, from the early evolution of the universe to the spiritual evolution of humans.

The Law of Necessity

Each of the stages of evolution consists of a unique principle of conscious energy (element, life, emotion, mind, wisdom, and love) with its own distinctive patterns of behavior. In a given species or person, each principle evolves only as far as is needed for the next principle to emerge, and each new principle appears out of absolute necessity. The full evolution of a given principle requires the appearance of the next one.

For example, heart and mind must be developed to a high degree before wisdom and love consciousness can develop. Also, every factor and experience in the evolution of the individual or species (including disease, death, good health, wealth, poverty, etc.) is present out of evolutionary necessity. This does not mean that we should not try to change our circumstances. The effort to do so contributes substantially to the evolution of consciousness. We are meant to struggle to improve ourselves. The effort develops our hidden capacities.

The Law of Integration

In the individual, the growth of the various energies is adjusted to maintain the integrity of the whole and to achieve the ultimate goal of evolution: the evolution of consciousness. What cannot be integrated is discarded. The three aspects of consciousness—knowledge, will, and feeling—are also mutually balanced and integrated as evolution proceeds. This is a continuous process, and at a given moment imbalance is often evident. Thus, usually we see people more developed in one area than in another. A scholar may be unable to feel deep emotion, or a person of intense emotion may be lacking in will. Because of this process of integration, "the balance of the entire being is shaken up gently every moment and every moment it is being recreated"[2] (p. 122).

The Law of Sacrifice

As suggested in the law of integration, each principle of conscious energy sacrifices its independent existence and nature so that the later principles can evolve. Plants are sacrificed for animals, and animals and plants for humans. Family and community life also depends upon the sacrifice of individual interests. Death is necessary so that life can continue.

The law of sacrifice helps explain the ill health that we see in the human species. Organic energy sacrifices the stability of the organism for the sake of mental development. As human culture moves from primarily agricultural to industrial and postindustrial, the incidence of chronic disease increases. The lifestyle of civilized humanity is less conducive to health than is an agricultural existence. Organic energy has paid the price of progress.

Often illness itself contributes to an evolution of heart, mind, and spirit. Numerous studies have confirmed this. One dramatic example of this law of sacrifice is Stephen Hawking. This brilliant theoretical physicist, paralyzed from the neck down, has done his work from the confines of a wheelchair. One wonders if he would have been so creative in his mental work if his body had been functioning normally. Among persons confronted with life-threatening illness, we often find an increased emphasis on values related to spirituality, friendship, and family.

The Law of Compressed Processes

The pace of evolution is increasing. This is possible because of the law of compressed processes. According to this law, every movement leaves an impression, or memory, that makes reproduction of the movement easier at each successive attempt. We see that the first time an action is taken, it is much more difficult to do than it is after many repetitions. The same is true in evolution. It took centuries for fish to evolve. But the human fetus goes through the entire evolutionary series in nine months, passing into and out of the fish form very quickly. In mental evolution, a child passes through all the centuries of humanity's development in a few years. Thus, today's children easily become computer literate whereas their grandparents take much more time to learn the same skills. Sheldrake[11], as we discussed earlier, maintains that this law of compressed processes is due to the existence of morphic fields. The 100th monkey phenomenon is just one example that illustrates this law.

CONCLUSION

We have surveyed our world from subatomic particles to ultimate reality in this attempt to establish a philosophical foundation for health and healing. Several key ideas that will inform subsequent chapters have been introduced. Most fundamental are the ideas that all energy is conscious and that the universe is made of conscious energy. The evolution of consciousness is the driving force behind the evolution of form. Each stage of evolution is marked by a dramatic shift into greater knowing, willing, and feeling. New principles emerge that support life, mind, and spirit. At the human level, the soul individuates and continues evolving through the mechanisms of reincarnation and karma. Several laws govern evolution: the law of necessity, the law of integration, the law of sacrifice, and the law of compressed processes. These laws will assume a central role in our discussion of health, illness, and healing.

CHAPTER 2

HEALTH

THE MEANING OF HEALTH

Health is closely related to the evolution of consciousness. True health is the constant development of greater knowledge-will-feeling at every level of conscious energy. One is healthy when all of one's energies are conscious and functioning to their full capacity and are also in harmony or equilibrium with each other. The evolutionary view of life provides a different perspective than usual on the concept of health. Health is not simply maintaining the status quo. It means increasing our capacity to know, will, and feel at every level. As our capacities increase, what it means to be healthy will change correspondingly. Each level of conscious energy manifests its own principles and characteristics and has its own characteristics of health.

Among all the dimensions of our being, those that emerged later in the course of evolution are more defining of our humanity than are those that we share with our animal ancestors. Heart, mind, and spirit make us human. These later evolutes of conscious energy are potentially more powerful and have the capacity to reorganize and reintegrate all the levels that came before them. Thus, when we look at the concept of health, we must give special emphasis to heart, mind, and spirit. Problems in any of these areas have the potential to result in physical disease.

We need to understand what proper functioning means, then, in each dimension of the person. Physical health brings strength and mobility. Organic health means the body's systems are successfully accomplishing the primary goal of life—self-preservation. This requires that each organ system carry out its function effectively and that all systems be well integrated. Emotional health is a condition of basic trust of self and others, the ability to give and receive affection, and the capacity to maintain long-term relationships that foster mutual growth. It means also the ability to acknowledge and express negative emotions in a constructive way.

Mental health requires a stable ego, a sense of self-worth, and self-confidence. A healthy mind can think rationally, can learn new ideas and express them clearly to others, and is able to solve new problems. A healthy mind is actively learning no matter what the person's age. A general sense of optimism (no matter what the circumstances) is also important for mental health. Later, we will look at the characteristics of high-level health—that is, when the spiritual dimension of the person integrates all other aspects into their highest potential.

Physical or organic needs and desires primarily drive some people's behavior, whereas others seem more motivated by emotional or mental satisfactions. Fewer people turn to spiritual sources for fulfillment. In this sense, the sportsman, the scholar, and the contemplative have little in common. In each of these, different centers of energy dominate behavior and personality. Can we say that any single center should outweigh the others in a healthy person? Is the Olympic athlete healthier than the theoretical physicist?

Remember our criteria of health: All systems should be functioning according to their nature and duty, and consciousness at each level of existence should be developing greater knowledge, will, and feeling. By these criteria, the athlete and the scholar may or may not be healthy. We cannot say automatically that one is healthier than the other is. Both might have found a way to nurture all dimensions of their selves. From an evolutionary point of view, however, a healthy person must be developing the capacities of heart, mind, and spirit.

By these criteria, then, a person with a diseased body will not necessarily be in poor health. A very dear friend recently died at age 38 of metastatic breast cancer. Lisa fought her cancer with all the medical resources available. At the same time, she worked on self-development in her relationships, her mental capacities, and her spirituality right until the day she died. She brought truth into her relationships and moved closer to those friends who wanted to help her grow during her illness. She studied vocabulary, world history, and speed-reading. She began to follow a spiritual path seriously and meditated twice daily without fail, no matter how ill she became. She died at peace and with great dignity. Lisa was an inspiring example of how a person can actually increase in health even when terminally ill. She transformed these abstract ideas into living reality.

The nature of health changes as a person evolves. What is healthy for a person at one stage of development is not healthy at a different stage. This is easy to see in the arena of child development. Though necessary for a neonate, it is not healthy for a six-year-old to stay in his or her mother's lap all day. In the evolutionary view, development does not end with adulthood. Each person has particular strengths and weaknesses and a unique path of evolution to follow. How can one know, then, what health is for oneself?

One must have an inner sense of one's capacities and limitations. Then the effort can be made to overcome one's limitations and fully develop one's capacities. In every arena one can ask, "Am I developing greater knowledge, a stronger will, and richer feeling? Am I balanced—or does one level of consciousness dominate to the detriment of others? Are the various aspects of my personality in harmony, or am I suffering from inner conflicts?" These are some inner checks that may help one assess the state of one's health.

OUR MULTIDIMENSIONAL CONSCIOUSNESS

We have seen that consciousness is present at each level of our being. Before we consider the possibility of the further evolution of consciousness, we should look at the current human condition. We will describe how knowledge, will, and feeling manifest at each level. The physical body can perceive mechanical, chemical, and electromagnetic stimuli. A person with an intact nervous system can feel pain and sometimes locate the source very precisely. Kinesthetic awareness—perception of the body's parts in relation to each other and to the environment—keeps a person upright. These are two examples of bodily knowing.

The body has a very strong will to survive and to live a full existence. Sick people often survive far beyond their expected life span, and athletes constantly break world records as they extend their bodies' limits. When a life-threatening situation demands it, a weak person can perform extraordinary acts of physical strength. Even in ordinary circumstances, there is a strong will to seek variety in sensory stimulation.

The body also feels, often very keenly. Pain is not only a chemical or mechanical stimulus. It creates a self-modification, or feeling, in the body. Endorphins are released. Anti-inflammatory chemicals rush to the site of injury. Pleasurable sensations likewise cause release of immune-building substances. Feelings of heat and cold, fatigue, vibration, and pressure also cause modifications in the body.

We have considered physical and organic consciousness together because they are inextricably integrated in the human body. Emotional consciousness is far more profound, subtle, and sensitive than the body. It can tune in to a beloved's heart across all barriers of space and time. The high vibrations of love can clear away all bodily ills. Likewise, negative emotions can lead to organic disease. Academic psychologists have only recently recognized the existence of emotional intelligence. Through very complex communications, we are able to know what others are actually feeling. This may, in fact, contradict what is being perceived physically through words. A mother may know that her child has been injured at the actual moment it happens, long before she is notified by school authorities. Deep emotion in its aspect of self-modification affects us in profound ways, bringing suffering or bliss into the heart.

The mind, we saw earlier, takes bodily perceptions and concepts gathered from the senses, amplifies them through the imagination, and molds them into abstract ideas and ideals. Scientific understanding is probing ever more deeply into the microcosm and macrocosm. The power of ideas is such that the entire course of history can change when they penetrate a population. Thoughts have an immense capacity for self-modification. For example, if someone believes he or she is dying, death may result even in the absence of disease. Hope, in turn, can bring life to someone on the threshold of death.

At the level of spiritual consciousness, we can perceive a reality that transcends space, time, ego, and all mental concepts. For some, this reality is experienced in nature, in moments of deep love, or in artistic inspiration. A profound peace and joy accompanies those moments when we are in tune with spiritual reality. This experience can transform the entire being and redirect life permanently.

These are the ordinary capacities of our multidimensional consciousness. We have defined health as the evolution of consciousness. So, in addition to looking at humanity's current state, we also need to examine human potentialities. Murphy[18] has compiled extensive evidence of what he calls the *human transformative capacity*. He identifies 12 classes and subclasses of extraordinary human functioning. He provides extensive documentation for each of the classes listed in Table 2–1.

It is significant that all of the higher capacities listed by Murphy can be subsumed within the tripartite consciousness of knowing-willing-feeling. Murphy is describing the evolution of consciousness. This comprehensive collection of data on human potential supports the thesis of evolving consciousness. Murphy[18] comments, "I firmly believe . . . that all of us can realize at least some of the extraordinary possibilities described here. I am convinced that men and women young and old, in widely disparate situations, at times experience the unitive awareness, selfless love, and redeeming joy that crown human life" (p. 6).

HIGH-LEVEL HEALTH

High-level health is present when the spiritual dimension of the person is vital and strong enough to integrate and harmonize all aspects of the being. A pervasive sense of well-being is present, even in the presence of physical disease. The senses function correctly, with minimal distortion from thoughts or desires. The body carries out its activities of maintenance, growth, repair, and reproduction without much stress or strain. The heart is stable and is not upset by negative emotions such as jealousy or anger. One can withstand loss and grief without disintegrating. Love, peace, and joy provide support even in difficult times.

In high-level health the mind is clear and is able to use reason and logic when needed, but it also draws upon intuition and direct insight. It can analyze a situation without prejudice. One's sense of self is intact and pervasive, yet not tinged by excessive egoism, for one is also supported by a sense of connection with all of humanity. The will is strong, but it is not used to harm others. There is an awareness of an underlying unity transcending the material universe. One feels a deep connection with this integrative reality, is supported by it, and lives in it.

The Sanskrit word for health—*svasthya*—reflects this vision of high-level health. This word also means "established in the Self." Notice the word *self* is capitalized in this definition. This is a translation of the Sanskrit word A*tman*,

TABLE 2–1   Murphy's Classification of Extraordinary Human Functioning

1. Perception of external events
   A. extraordinary sensory perception
   B. clairvoyance or remote viewing
   C. perceptions of entities or events outside the normally perceivable world
2. Somatic awareness and self-regulation
   A. extraordinary somatic awareness mediated by the central nervous system
   B. extraordinary somatic awareness mediated by internal clairvoyance
3. Communication abilities
   A. extraordinary communication abilities mediated by sensory cues
   B. extraordinary communication abilities mediated by telepathic interaction
4. Vitality
5. Movement abilities
   A. extraordinary physical movement
   B. levitation
   C. out-of-body experience
   D. movement into other worlds
6. Abilities to alter the environment
   A. extraordinary hand-eye coordination and dexterity
   B. extrasomatic influence upon the environment
7. Pain and pleasure
8. Cognition
   A. mystical knowledge
   B. scientific, artistic, and philosophic inspiration
9. Volition
10. Individuation and sense of self
    A. ego-transcendent identity
    B. cognitive-emotional-behavioral uniqueness
11. Love
12. Bodily structures, states, and processes

which means the universal self, as opposed to *atman*, or individual self. When one is established in the self, then, one identifies with all. One is in love with the divinity in all. As we discussed earlier, it is not human love that brings this state of total peace and joy. Human love prepares us, however, for this ultimate experience.

THE HUMAN ENERGY SYSTEM

Because everything is made of conscious energy, and energy consists of vibrations, we can visualize each principle of conscious energy as vibrating within a certain frequency range, much like the stations on a radio. The higher frequency vibrations, or simply the higher vibrations, are more powerful than the lower ones. X-rays are a good example of this. The visible range of frequencies is quite low on the energy spectrum. X-rays, though not visible, are much higher frequency than is light and can do much more harm, as well as much good when used therapeutically. Similar is the situation within the person.

An individual is a complex field of vibrations of many different frequencies. In the average person, more often than not, these physical, organic, emotional, mental, and spiritual vibrations are not in harmony. Perfect health is when all of the vibrations of one's being are in harmony, or equilibrium. We will examine how this can be possible. But first we will look at how the various energies of the human being are organized.

Classical Indian spiritual doctrine[1, 4] describes the structure and organization of the various energies that make up a human being. There is said to be an invisible chain of energy centers very near the spinal column, beginning at the base of the spine and ending at the top of the head. This is called *kundalini*. The energy in each center moves slowly in the pattern of a wheel. Each center is called a *chakra*—the Sanskrit word for "wheel."

There is a center corresponding to each of the principles of conscious energy that have evolved—physical, organic, emotional, mental, and spiritual. The vibrations from each of these centers are responsible for the complex activity and behavior that is manifest in human life. As consciousness evolves in the person, different centers vibrate more intensely and exert more influence on the other centers. Genes therefore are not the primary determinants of physical characteristics and behavior. They are the vehicles of expression of these energy centers.

How do these centers of energy actually influence each other and evolve? Ramananda[4] addresses this subject. The energy centers are concentrated at specific points along the spinal column. Each center has an upper and a lower pole. The lower pole is strongly connected with and influenced by the center below, and the same is true of the upper pole. In this sense, we can speak of *lower emotions* and *higher emotions*. Lower emotions are strongly connected with organic vibrations, and higher emotions are more connected with thoughts (mental vibrations).

For example, jealousy and anger are most often rooted in organic cravings such as sexual desires. Higher emotions such as universal love and sympathy transcend organic needs and arise from values and ideals. The vibrations of the lower pole of an energy center cause the vibrations of the higher pole of the next lowest center to vibrate at a frequency closer to their own. This sympathetic vibration is much like the strings of a guitar that vibrate in response to other vibrating strings nearby.

The same relationship holds for the higher pole of a center and the lower pole of the next highest center. As the person evolves, the dominant energy center moves higher up the spinal column. Thus, the vibrations of all the other centers are adjusted accordingly. Vibrations that are not in harmony with the new center of energy gradually decline and eventually cease. There is a progressive increase in the frequency of vibrations, corresponding with a gradual growth from a physically rooted consciousness to a mental and spiritual consciousness.

The structure of the human energy centers has been secret knowledge among Indian spiritual masters for thousands of years. Its direct manipulation remains secret. But a natural, slow refinement and evolution of these centers can take place in the course of a lifetime and will result in the evolution of the person's consciousness. There are measures that can aid in this process— moderation in food and sex, regular gentle exercise such as yoga, and reducing anxiety and stress in one's daily life. Certain forms of meditation may substantially accelerate the upward movement of these energies.

The vibrations emanating from the environment also directly influence one's centers of energy through the mechanism described above. They can either aid or hinder the evolution of one's consciousness. One can seek out friends whose interests, behavior, and temperaments stimulate one's own growth. One can also spend time in environments that are specially endowed with high vibrations. Every continent has sacred places that are preserved for the uplift of humanity. In every setting, one can pay attention to the energies in the atmosphere and be selective about where one spends time.

Thus, each person is a field of vibrating energy centers, each center regulating its respective principle of conscious energy. These centers influence each other, as well, and respond to outside vibrations. Good health depends upon a continual reestablishment of equilibrium among these centers, as they are constantly evolving at varying speeds.

In general, the higher frequency vibrations of heart, mind, and spirit should exert a strong regulating influence on the physical and organic energies. However, usually the opposite is true. Often, a person uses logic and reason to justify physical or emotional cravings. Objectivity is lost, and the mind accepts the slavery of unhealthy needs. This is possible because physical and emotional energies are older and more entrenched than the newcomer, mind. They are preestablished powers, and mind must evolve to a high degree before it can establish its rule. In the average person, we find varying degrees of struggle going on among these competing principles, each of which has its own agenda.

There is also a lack of equilibrium in the evolution of body, heart, and mind in the individual. Body, heart, and mind develop at different rates. There is a constant effort to reestablish equilibrium, so that there is a natural tendency for the personality to experience disorder. The mind advances, and the heart is left behind. Thus, the heart races to catch up and outpaces mind for a time.

Each person goes through many cycles of uneven development throughout life. The healthier person will be able to modulate this unevenness so that the personality does not disintegrate. Mental illness is characterized by a severe disorganization in which the various energies of the person are exceedingly unbalanced. Adolescence is a time of rapid development, and varying degrees of instability are almost inevitable. This is why adolescence is so full of turbulence and awkwardness. Stability and a more even growth herald the onset of maturity.

The root cause of this unevenness is the lack of an equalizing factor. Mind should be up to this task, but it starts out weak and, when strong, its control can be stifling to growth. Mind has no heart and does not value the needs of the body. Its knowledge is limited, as we discussed in chapter 1. Unnatural suppressions of heart and body dictated by fears of hell or of social approbation cause great harm to the personality. Suppressed needs and desires eventually rise up with a vengeance. It requires a consciousness more tolerant than the mind to integrate and equalize our energies.

Fortunately, there is a way out. As discussed in chapter 1, human beings have the potential to develop greater wisdom and love. In one lifetime, the ordinary person will not achieve these completely. However certainly in one lifetime our consciousness can be cleansed, strengthened, and refined. We can experience interludes of true insight, wisdom, and perhaps even love. With this process we may eventually attain a high level of health.

TRUTHFUL LIVING

Health is present when all dimensions of the person are functioning according to their highest potential. This is what we mean by *truthful living*. An organism performing all its functions in truth is a healthy organism. Truth is the natural manifestation of the individual. Truthful living is being one's true self. Fear of criticism or desire of approval loses its grip. This requires that one know and express oneself. Of course, this does not mean that there is no effort to change. A healthy person is always trying to learn and grow. Truthful living also is living in harmony with nature as much as possible. The truthful life becomes simple and natural.

Making one's life simple and natural is the art of living. This does not mean that one must move to the country and become a farmer. Even in the largest city one can bring simplicity into life and live in harmony with nature. Nature is full of rhythms. A natural life is regular in its habits and routines. Creating a daily routine is very helpful. One may object that routine makes life less natural, more artificial. A careful look at the natural world easily dispels this misconception. Nature operates according to rhythms organized into biological routines. Creating daily routines is very helpful. You may object that routine denaturalizes life. But look carefully at the natural world. It is full of rhythms, organized into biological routines. Seasons come in their own time and in order. Animals and plants live in cycles of activity and rest. Our own bodies have similar innate rhythms that we should listen to and support. Awakening and sleeping at the same time every day is a first step. The closer these times can match sunrise and sunset times, the better. The body follows circadian rhythms of day and night. Following these rhythms will bring greater stability and energy. An irregular sleep-wake cycle is considered a risk factor for health problems.

Another step toward simplicity and natural living is an eating routine that is regular in content and timing. Many people find this enormously difficult. The pleasure of eating seems to be dependent on variety and unpredictability. But eating either much more or much less than normal or eating a totally different type of meal creates fatigue and can even dull one's mind. A regular routine of eating will help maintain a stable level of energy and function.

What one eats should also be as natural as possible. It is preferable to eliminate, or at least reduce, processed foods and meat from the diet. Humans have the teeth of vegetarians, not of carnivores. Whole grains, fresh fruits and vegetables, nuts, legumes, and a moderate amount of dairy products will sustain the body without clogging the arteries.

A routine of sleeping and eating automatically puts one in harmony with the rhythms of nature. Rather than limiting freedom, it actually provides more time and energy to work and play. Less time and energy go into making decisions about what or when to eat and catching up on sleep.

Ultimately, living truthfully means living in harmony with the universe. The universe functions in cycles. All things with form must change form. There is no permanence in form. We get attached to the forms that surround us—friends, family, and loved ones—and resist their change. It is healthy to be able to accept change that is inevitable. This is the truth of our universe. When it is time to let go, we should try to surrender to the rhythms of life and death, to the winds of change.

Bringing truth into one's relationships also can improve health. This is difficult for many people. Intimate relationships are often built either on illusions or on unfilled needs. Unsatisfied with what they really are, one may either feign happiness or try to mold the other to create a person more to one's liking. Truthful relationships are based on mutual honesty and acceptance. Bringing truth into one's relationships will promote a higher level of health by reducing the strain associated with maintaining false appearances.

Truth of the senses is another characteristic of health. The senses become dulled or confused when they are not used correctly. They provide misleading input. Harmful foods taste good. Crude images look appealing. Harsh sounds bring pleasure. Modern Western culture encourages abuse of the senses. Eventually the senses lose their sensitivity and sensibility. The stage is set for ill health when the senses no longer can discriminate between life-affirming and life-negating experience.

Bringing truth back into the senses requires that one restore their discrimination. It helps to withdraw whatever has been distorting them—for example, if a person usually consumes a diet high in salt, he or she can eliminate salt completely for several days and then reintroduce it in small amounts. A more moderate amount of salt will then satisfy his or her tongue. Fasting for several days may help to readjust a person's pattern of excessive food consumption. The senses are the organs of perception and the foundation of knowledge, and they are vitally important to the evolution of consciousness. We need to sharpen our sensory capacities, but overloading them does not do this. Using them correctly will.

CREATING HEALTHY HABITS

We are creatures of habit. Habits mold individual and group behavior. One should carefully examine one's habits to see if they are promoting health or harming it. This means not only physical habits like smoking, drinking alcohol or caffeinated beverages, exercise, and fat intake. Emotional, mental, and spiritual habits are potentially even more influential on health. Healthy habits can be cultivated for each level of conscious energy.

Physical Habits

Physical habits are clearly the foundation of health. We explored earlier how sleep and dietary habits can put one in harmony with nature's rhythms. The habit of physical exercise is equally important. Many of our modern chronic illnesses—Type II diabetes, hypertension, high cholesterol, heart disease, certain cancers, and arthritis—are either caused by, correlated with, or significantly worsened by physical inactivity. The modern lifestyle, full of conveniences to save time and effort, creates sedentary living.

It takes deliberate planning and effort, therefore, to ensure that one obtains adequate exercise. As with any healthy routine, determination and commitment are required. Gentle stretching, rhythmic movement, and aerobic activity should all be part of an exercise program. Weight bearing is also necessary to maintain bone strength.

Changing physical habits requires a strong will. Some people find that they can only change habits if they never again engage in whatever behavior they are trying to change. Others find that an occasional indulgence makes the change easier to manage. It is always helpful to have a supportive environment for the change. This means not only social support, but also modifications in the physical environment that make it easier to maintain the newly developing habit—for example, removing all of a harmful food from the house.

One can sometimes trick an unhealthy system into thinking it is healthy by changing its habits. Then it may actually become healthier. For example, a 42-year-old patient with advanced cardiomyopathy was a candidate for a heart transplant. After learning of his condition 3 years ago, he insisted on carrying out his usual activities, taking care only not to exert himself to the point of causing shortness of breath. He refused to go to bed and wait to die. His cardiac function is now better than when he was diagnosed.

Emotional and Mental Habits

Changing negative emotional and thought patterns into positive, health-promoting attitudes requires enormous effort. Automatic emotional reactions often are inappropriate in a situation and can cause serious problems. Deeply ingrained ways of thinking can close one's mind to other points of view. These form the roots of prejudice. Forming premature judgments of people and situations is another harmful habit of the mind.

Emotional attachment is a deeply ingrained human habit. In spiritual teachings throughout the world, much emphasis is given to the importance of loosening one's attachments. Attachment is being stuck to someone. Attachment forms the foundation of family life. There are many theories about how to facilitate attachment between a mother and newborn. Clearly, at certain stages of development, attachment is necessary. But, as consciousness evolves, attachments naturally lessen. One expands one's range of association, first from parents to mate or spouse, then to one's children, and finally beyond family ties to larger social groups.

Ultimately, a consciousness that is evolving in a healthy manner will begin to identify with the entire human family—and even with the entire universe. Family gossip will come from international newswires. The earth itself will be home. The field of transpersonal ecology promotes this sense of connection with all of nature. It will be impossible to exploit or destroy the natural world when we feel it is our true home. It will be impossible to wage war on other nations if we feel they are family.

Outgrowing attachments does not mean abandoning relationships. In fact, it means that relationships are strengthened as they become established in truth. The truth is that all human relationships end at the moment of death. It is also true that we are connected to every person on the face of the earth. This is more apparent than ever in the global economy, as the fortunes of all nations rise and fall together.

Nonattachment is being ready to establish truth in one's relationships. If problems exist, they are acknowledged. One is ready to change emotional patterns in order to solve the problems. If one is attached, one resists change. Nonattachment means also opening one's heart to all people, not saving love only for immediate family or old friends. These characteristics of nonattachment are signs of increasing emotional health and of the evolution of consciousness. The goal is to establish a love habit that extends to all, not only a few.

Many mental habits also interfere with growth. Mental laziness is a common problem. The computer revolution has exacerbated this tendency. One no longer needs to work out a math problem in the mind. There is a calculator.

Web sites are replacing books. Information can be gotten with ease. This is not bad in itself. What really matters is what we do with information. Despite the opinion of many in digital research, information is not equivalent to knowledge, and it is even further from wisdom.

Using the mind well is like exercising a muscle. One needs to use it every day in order to keep it functioning optimally. Reading books and newspapers, studying a new subject, or learning a language will keep the mind active and exploring. This is an important step toward health. Even if one is confined to bed or unable to move, the mind should stay active and engaged.

Changing mental habits requires a very strong will and constant vigilance to catch negative emotions or thoughts when they commence. Developing a repertoire of counterthoughts is helpful. One can formulate positive feelings and thoughts, perhaps even in writing, so that they can be available at the first sign of negativity. If this proves difficult to accomplish on one's own, there are numerous books that provide a source of positive and encouraging sentiments to supplant self-defeating thoughts.

Spiritual Habits

Maintaining a spiritual routine is another habit that can be of great value in improving health. The wisdom and experience of the ages suggests that meditation is a simple and very effective means of nurturing one's spiritual center. It tunes one's higher consciousness into the subtler vibrations of the universe.

Meditation means different things to different people. For some, it is synonymous with relaxation. For others, it means emptying the mind. My personal experience is of filling the mind with high vibrations and invoking the higher vibrations of the cosmos to come into myself. Not only the mind is filled; the entire being can be flooded with spiritual energy. When one invokes the highest frequency vibrations into one's system, they enter through the top of the head. This descent of cosmic energy sets up a new order of vibration throughout the entire being. A chain reaction of accelerating frequencies is set up.

Invoking cosmic energy can be done in many ways. Prayer is one means. Mantra is another. *Mantra* is a single word or phrase, repeated usually throughout the entire meditation. A mantra is a special, energy-endowed sound. The source of the energy of the mantra will determine how powerful it is. There are ancient mantras that are so powerful that they can radically transform one's life. These are sacred syllables, or names of the supreme reality or its aspects. The ancient mantras are handed down from one practitioner to the next in an unbroken chain of transmission. One is fortunate to find such an adherent of the mantra. Most people must do without. In the meantime, one can choose a word or phrase that has some special personal meaning and power and repeat it in meditation.

Meditating at sunrise and sunset—called *sandhya dhyana* in Sanskrit—is the most ancient spiritual tradition known. It puts one in harmony with the rhythms of the natural world. The energy of the earth is special at these times. This routine is invaluable in establishing and maintaining high-level health.

Some forms of meditation (commonly called *kundalini yoga*) attempt to raise the level of vibration of all the centers starting from the lowest center, rather than from the highest. This creates an ascent, rather than a descent, of energy. These practices can be harmful. The organic energy unleashed can cause sudden and severe disintegration of the personality.

CONCLUSION

We have explored the meaning of health in its most comprehensive sense. First, we examined the structure of the human energy system and found it to be multidimensional, consisting of physical, organic, emotional, mental, and spiritual levels of consciousness. We described the normal consciousness of each level of energy and also looked at Murphy's schema for classifying extraordinary human capacities. Based on this examination of ordinary and extraordinary consciousness, we were able to define high-level health, the state when the spiritual dimension of the person is integrating and harmonizing all aspects of the being. High-level health is possible because the structure of the human energy system facilitates mutual influence among all the centers of energy and is open to the influence of cosmic and local environmental vibrations. Truthful living, we found, is living in harmony with the cosmos and is the natural manifestation of the individual. We explored how truth is expressed at each level of consciousness. Next, we discussed how to establish healthy habits at each level of conscious energy.

We ended with a discussion of how to establish a spiritual routine so that all other aspects of life can be put in order. The insights and suggestions put forth in this chapter are all distilled from ancient spiritual and healing traditions. Keeping a healthy routine is the foundation of true health, and this foundation has always been considered to be at the spiritual level. The universe operates in rhythms, and we are no exception. If we put order and balance into life and establish a routine, we will find freedom to blossom into our true selves.

CHAPTER 3

AN EVOLUTIONARY VIEW OF ILLNESS

INTRODUCTION

Conscious energy is self-organizing. It spontaneously forms structures and, through them, adopts certain functions. Disease is a disturbance in the structure or function of the physical or organic level of consciousness. Illness is the set of symptoms, behaviors, emotions, and attitudes that result in a feeling of unwellness. Illness can occur at any level of consciousness. This means that one can be ill without having a disease. One can also have a disease and not be ill.

DISEASE

Scientists have been able to describe the structure and function of energy at the physical and organic levels with great precision. They are dissecting units of energy into smaller and smaller parts so that now we are examining subatomic particles and genes. This effort to break the body down into its smallest possible parts is characteristic of the mechanistic view of disease. Mechanism treats the body as if it were a machine. It believes that disease is due to some external agent that disrupts the physical or chemical reactions taking place in the body. The signs and symptoms of a disease are thought to be due to these deranged reactions and serve no useful purpose. Mechanistic medicine tries to suppress the symptoms and remove the disease-causing agent. Dramatic advances in mechanistic medicine have been made at the molecular and genetic levels. Designer drugs are able to target the altered chemical processes involved in diseases such as arthritis, Alzheimer's dementia, cancer, and hypertension.

But advances in mechanistic medicine should not hinder our search for the deeper causes of disease. We must recognize the limitations of the mechanistic view. These limitations are apparent when we survey the major causes of morbidity and mortality in Western developed societies. Cancer, heart disease, diabetes, alcoholism, and stroke are all clearly multifactorial in causation. They are not readily explained by the mechanistic model. We can identify the cellular changes that are associated with these diseases. However, we cannot explain completely why some people are stricken and others are not, and why some are able to live long, productive lives despite having a major chronic illness.

An alternative perspective on the roots of disease is based on the philosophy of vitalism, also known as *organicism*. Organicism recognizes the molecular correlates of disease but incorporates them within a broader framework. Organicism maintains that a different form of energy organizes physical and chemical interactions into the processes that support life. Within our framework, this energy is called *organic energy*, which we discussed in Chapter 1. Here we want to apply the basic principles that govern organic energy to our understanding of disease.

Recall that the fundamental driving force of organic energy is the will to live. It has a stunning intelligence that only becomes more impressive as we understand more deeply how it operates at the molecular level. Given the highly effective consciousness that is present in organic energy, we must examine the usual medical approach to disease management. Mechanistic medicine assumes that the symptoms of disease should be suppressed. That is, fever should be brought down, discharges should be dried up, vomiting should be controlled, and diarrhea should be stopped. These symptoms make the patient uncomfortable or can even cause harm. Patients expect to leave the medical office with a pill that will alleviate their discomfort.

The organicist philosophy maintains that the symptoms of disease are a result of organic energy's highly intelligent effort to heal the body. Fever kills bacteria. Discharges and diarrhea eliminate toxic organisms or products from the body. "Symptoms, then, are part of a constructive phenomenon that is the best 'choice' the organism can make, given the circumstances."[36]

Symptoms develop in two ways. The first and most common is as described above, when they originate in the organism's well-orchestrated healing response. In this case, the therapeutic effort should be to stimulate and support this response, rather than to suppress the symptoms. The second way that symptoms occur is when a body function is disrupted from a pathological process or external agent. Genetic disorders, tumors, major trauma, and overwhelming infection fit this description. Here, mechanistic medicine may justifiably suppress the organism's natural response in order to save life. Unfortunately, often it does this too well, as in the case of cancer chemotherapy, which normally suppresses the body's own immune system.

Using the definition of consciousness set forth in Chapter 1, we can describe and classify health problems as disorders of consciousness at any of its levels. We can develop a taxonomy of illness that ranges from the physical to the spiritual levels of consciousness. Table 3–1 presents an attempt to create such a taxonomy.

Table 3–1 shows that there is some overlap, as well as intimate interconnections, among the various levels of consciousness.

TABLE 3–1

	Physical	Organic	Emotional	Mental	Spiritual
Acute problems	Injuries; infections; electrolyte imbalances	Acute inflammation; infections; allergic reactions	Depression; aggressive behavior; grief	Delirium; psychotic episodes; acute anxiety	Existential crisis; crisis of faith; spiritual emergency
Chronic problems	Degenerative diseases	Addictions; immune disorders (e.g., cancer, autoimmune disease) inflammatory diseases (e.g., asthma); endocrine disorders; chronic infections	Bipolar affective disorder; violence	Neuroses; anxiety disorders; psychoses; dementia	Alienation; hopelessness; loss of faith

In dealing with illness, it is most effective to correct chemical or other physical derangements at the highest possible level of energy. By highest we mean, as explained in Chapter 1, the level that is vibrating at a more subtle, higher frequency. The question arises whether all physical problems ultimately are rooted in spiritual disorders, because the spiritual level is the most subtle and powerful. It does not appear to be the case, however, because even spiritually realized beings are subject to disease and death. (Disease in a spiritual person, in such cases, can be inherent in the genes that are karmically inherited. See Chapter 1 on karma). Organic energy does appear to have a built-in biological clock that eventually runs down. As discussed earlier, this is an absolutely essential feature of life.

Disease, in most cases, is a vitiation of organic-level energy. This level has greater knowledge, will, and feeling than does the physical level and is therefore usually both the source of disease and the source of healing. However, the ultimate cause may be in a higher level than the organic. Emotional, mental, or even spiritual disequilibrium often results in disease on the physical or organic level.

For example, diabetes is due to an imbalance in either the production or utilization of insulin. On a macroscopic level, it is due to an imbalance in activity— lack of exercise is a significant risk factor for Type II diabetes. Depression may be due to an overly sensitive emotionality or to a deficit in serotonin, a neurotransmitter secreted in the brain. Similarly, psychosis may have its roots in an imbalanced personality or in a biochemical imbalance in the brain. The cure of a disease requires that the imbalance that caused it be corrected. Treating the symptoms will not provide a cure.

As we showed in the case of diabetes, the underlying imbalance may be present on more than one level. In this case, it will be most helpful to correct the imbalance at the highest, most broad level possible. So, increasing exercise will be a more effective solution to diabetes than will be taking drugs to stimulate insulin production or utilization. It causes a change in organic energy and does more benefit than its normally known physical effects. Exercise allows a freer flow of organic energy. Organic energy can fool the body into believing that it is normal again.

DISEASE AND EVOLUTION

From the evolutionary perspective, disease is a friend in one's evolutionary journey. It is an indicator of disequilibrium or imbalance. If one gives it due attention and tries to understand the message that it brings, disease can inspire change and accelerate the entire process of personal evolution. Recall our discussion of chaos and evolution in Chapter 1. Disease is a form of chaos. The person on the edge of chaos—that is, with a disease—has the opportunity to accelerate his or her personal evolution. An example will help illustrate this.

An overworked business executive who suffers a heart attack is forced to look at his lifestyle—at what he eats, how and when he eats, at his lack of exercise, at his intolerable level of stress, at his neglect of his wife and children. If he is smart, he will turn away from this life in which work is everything. He will see the connection between his lack of balance and his diseased heart. He will use the heart attack as a pivot for radical change. He will begin to live his life according to a different set of values. He may say, years later, "This is strange, but my heart attack was the best thing that ever happened to me!"

We observe a similar phenomenon in people who experience other life-threatening illnesses, such as HIV or cancer. Many studies have been conducted that document the transformative power of serious illness. I conducted a study of cancer patients in 1985. A dominant theme among patients I interviewed was the positive change in outlook and values that occurred after the diagnosis. Quality of life in many ways actually increased despite substantial physical suffering. Relationships were strengthened and behavior changed to reflect a new focus on transcendent values such as love, family, and friendship. Material values declined in importance. This and many other studies, most recently by Johnston-Taylor[37], support the thesis that serious disease has the ability to inspire transformative evolutionary change.

In many cases, a physical problem is a manifestation of a problem at a deeper (or higher) level of consciousness. For example, a patient has had a lifelong aversion to physical work. Along with this, she is extremely rigid in her habits. She does not like to do things differently than her usual routine. She has a brilliant mind but misuses it in worrying over tiny details of life. Given this background, it is understandable that she develops rheumatoid arthritis. The rigidity and aversion to work in her mind finds expression in rigid, dysfunctional joints.

The practitioner who treats this woman only on the physical level will never succeed in really healing her. She may take designer drugs to control the inflammation of her joints. However, without a change in her emotional and mental consciousness, the roots of her disease will not be touched. It may be too late for her to reverse the physical damage in her joints. But the effort of changing her emotional and mental outlook should not be abandoned, for her arthritis will certainly cause her joints to deteriorate further if these attitudes are not corrected.

Most people consider disease to be an utterly useless affront to their life and do everything they can to avoid it. When they are stricken with disease, they try every possible treatment, often including harmful drugs to suppress their symptoms. An evolutionary healer will gently guide the patient into an awareness of his or her imbalances and will suggest ways of gaining greater equilibrium. The healer will help the person listen to the messages brought by disease.

If a disease can be easily cured or runs a benign, self-limiting course, such as in the case of the common cold, how does it serve as a call for readjustment? The common cold offers an excellent example. Most people who catch a cold are under excessive stress, either physical, emotional, or mental, at the time. There is some imbalance in their life. The cold forces them to rest and relax. If they do not, then it becomes something more serious, like walking pneumonia, or a severe sinus infection, or bronchitis. A smart person who is in tune with his or her body will learn to recognize that state in which a cold develops in time to correct it and prevent the cold.

KARMA AND DISEASE

We have seen that disease is a result of an imbalance or maladjustment in physical or organic energy and that often it is due to emotional, mental, or even spiritual disequilibrium. But we still have not asked why disease occurs at all. Why is the world designed so that people become ill? Is perfect health a realistic possibility for the average person? From the evolutionary view, disease is both necessary and inevitable. It is necessary because it is an indicator of our inner state and inspires us to change, to strive for greater balance. It is inevitable because perfect equilibrium among all levels of consciousness is possible only when one has completed the evolutionary journey and reaches the highest level of evolution—love.

Ultimately, the law of karma governs one's state of health and the diseases that one acquires. The circumstances in which one finds oneself are often a response to our actions from previous lives. They are not punishment; they serve an educative role, teaching lessons necessary for one's growth.

This does not mean that one should not attempt to heal one's diseases. One of the lessons of serious illness is learning how to draw upon the best inner and outer resources that are available. One learns to ask questions and to challenge the authority of physicians. One learns to seek information on one's own and to take responsibility for our own treatment decisions. One learns to trust what one's own instincts might be telling one about the best course of treatment. It is critically important to learn these lessons. This is exactly how consciousness develops its capacity to know, feel, and will. However, sometimes a disease causes such drastic changes in structure or function that it cannot be reversed. This will happen only in accordance with the law of karma—that is, only if it's of absolute evolutionary necessity for the individual.

Karma uses various mechanisms to carry out its purpose. Genes are one of them. A soul will take birth in a particular body with a particular set of genes because of its karmic imperative. Whatever diseases are needed for a soul's evolution will be programmed into its genes. The discoveries of genetic medicine provide us with important insight into the ingenious manner in which karma actually accomplishes its task.

Efforts to change the course of disease through genetic manipulation—or any other medical treatment—are also part of the evolutionary process. Nothing said previously is meant to imply in any way that one we should not try to ameliorate diseases. One must make a full effort to do so. At the same time, one needs also to examine what role any current behaviors may have in either causing or maintaining the disease. But one also should recognize that the cause of a disease may be from a previous life of which there is no recollection.

The evolutionary process has deliberately made one's past lives inaccessible to our consciousness. It would be too confusing and not particularly helpful to remember past lives. It is hard enough to cope with the demands and lessons that one's present life brings. In rare cases, when there is a genuine remembrance of one's past life, it happens without any effort. There is no useful purpose served by reincarnation therapy.

Illness

Illness is the set of symptoms, behaviors, emotions, and attitudes that are associated with a feeling of unwellness. Suffering is due to the experience of illness, not to the disease itself. Illness is characterized by a lack of inner peace, a sense of pessimism, and/or an inability or unwillingness to carry out one's ordinary life functions. One feels unwell. A person who actually has a serious— even life-threatening—disease may show no signs of illness. The opposite is also true. A person can be ill but have no disease, at least on the physical or organic level.

Illness, however, often does contribute to the development and progression of disease. Body and mind are so intimately connected that change in either one will have repercussions in the other. Ramananda[4] gives several examples: "Physical illness brings disappointment and sadness to the mind. Physical weakness often makes people irritable. . . . Sorrow tires the body. Fear makes appetite disappear. Through anger it is possible to get fever and be stuck to a bed. Enthusiasm brings new energy to the body" (p. 109).

The framework set forth in Chapter 1 explains how the body-mind connection actually operates. Recall that all energy is conscious. The body, then, is conscious and, therefore, is innately responsive to the vibrations of thoughts and emotions. The vibrations of the spirit are even more powerful. Prayer has now been scientifically demonstrated to have an influence on physical conditions—even when the beneficiary has no awareness of being prayed for.[38] Distance poses no barrier to emotions, thoughts, or prayers. Even in the world of quantum particles, action at a distance is a known phenomenon.

Life-threatening illness has a profound potential to accelerate the evolution of consciousness. We can understand its power by examining the common hindrances to personal evolution. Ramananda[3] identifies three main obstacles: attachment, ego, and desire. In a child, these three qualities serve an important purpose. Without them, there is no drive to gather broader and more intense experience. But in a mature person, these same qualities become hindrances to personal evolution. They separate the individual from others, confine him or her to a small sphere of interest and relations, and lead to imbalances in personality.

A mature individual needs to loosen strong, exclusive attachments in order to cultivate a more universal affiliation. The wall of ego must be penetrated. Desire is best replaced by a sense of responsibility and sobriety. Wisdom should become the basis for action, and love—concern for the well-being of all—his or her ultimate motivation. Life-threatening illness forces a person to anticipate the severing of attachments, the bowing down of the ego, and the abandonment of desires. Ramananda[3] describes the profound impact of physical suffering:

> "Suffering, in whatever way it comes, deepens our consciousness. Man comes to have a wider and more sober view of the world than he has otherwise. He learns to bow. I have seen haughty heads bowing down when they have lain helpless in sickbeds. It is such a corrective! Prolonged sickness does not only over-haul the body. It over-hauls the mind as well. In the heat of strength we run roughshod over others, not knowing the wounds we inflict and the pains we cause. We know them when we lie in bed, a picture of utter helplessness. Then, we can appreciate the meaning of love and service. Then we know gentleness. Suffering teaches what no sermons or books can. It teaches what even prolonged meditation and worship cannot. It has a unique place in evolution!" (pp. 37–38).

ILLNESS AT VARIOUS LEVELS OF CONSCIOUSNESS

Physical Illness

As indicated in Table 3–1, purely physical illness is due primarily to injury or to acute infection contracted from the environment. This appears fairly straightforward. But even in the case of physical illness there often are other factors that are implicated in the chain of causation. An accident-prone person may have a problem with inattentiveness, for example, which is a mental deficit. An injured female treated in the emergency room may be a victim of domestic violence in a relationship that is deeply unhealthy.

Perhaps it is at the physical level that karmic factors hold particular relevance, for there may be no other obvious reason for a person to have fallen ill or be injured. A freak accident that leaves a person paralyzed for life is one example of a situation in which karma plays a major role. From the evolutionary point of view, everything happens for a reason, and the reason is often karmic. Karmically related incidents do have their roots in one's organic being and in the environment. They work through the genetic vehicle as do other normal happenings.

Organic Illness

Organic illness may be caused by addictions to sex, tobacco, alcohol, and certain foods. The organism begins to crave the experience these provide. This eventually creates havoc in the organism and subverts its primary goal of self-preservation. How does an organism's sense of what is healthy and not healthy become perverted? This is a complex issue. The immediate, overt pleasure brought by an addictive substance clouds the organism's perception of the covert damage being done. The addiction may serve as a substitute for a compelling psychological need that is stronger than the organic will to live.

All of the major physiological subsystems of the human organism are maintained by organic energy. The neuroendocrine system is the central regulating force of the organism and is a direct extension of organic energy. The immune and neuroendocrine systems are strongly connected with each other and with every other system, so that immune and neuroendocrine disorders have profound and extensive implications. In turn, the neuroendocrine system has links with mental and emotional consciousness. The neuroendocrine system is, in a sense, the linchpin of health. Disorders of the neuroendocrine system, then, can result in illness at virtually any level of consciousness.

Emotional Illness

The cause of most emotional illness can be found in excessive attachment or in the inability to love. The two go together. *Attachment* means taking to be one's own that which is not one's own, wanting to possess it forever. It is rooted in personal desires. As we discussed in Chapter 2, attachment is inherently resistant to change. Because change is inevitable, attachment brings intense emotional suffering. Children grow up and leave home. Spouses lose their health and beauty; they grow old and die. Friends do likewise. The more one is attached to these relationships, the more one will suffer.

It may seem a contradiction that attachment and an inability to love go together. We often think that the more attached one is to family and loved ones, the more love is present. But the love that we are aspiring to in the effort to advance our evolution is not possessive, not demanding, not meeting our self-centered desires. Instead, this love is self-fulfilling; it is happiest when the object of love is happy and well, regardless of whether that object is near or far. It respects the individuality of its beloved and is satisfied just to be in love. Further, the love that we seek is not exclusive to any one person or thing. It is universal, like the sun shining on all. It knows that it does not own anyone and that change and loss are inevitable. It is not by any means indifferent or cold; but it is ready to let go when the time comes.

The primary source of emotional illness is the inability to love—to give love. People who are emotionally ill often complain about the lack of love in their lives, as if receiving love is the problem. The root problem, however, is in giving love. If one is able to give love, then one automatically fulfills the need for love.

Depression is a widespread illness in modern industrialized societies. It is a complex problem and clearly has neurochemical correlates in the brain. For some people, it appears to have no external precipitants whatsoever. We call this *endogenous* or *major* depression. One can be depressed even in paradise. Karma, again, provides insight into this phenomenon.

But often depression occurs in response to an external condition or event. Even environmental conditions like lack of sunlight can lead to depression in a susceptible individual. Depression in response to an external loss—for example, the loss of a loved one—is a very common illness. Understanding the nature of attachment and love may be somewhat helpful in dealing with this state, but it is largely a condition that must be allowed to resolve itself with time. (Kubler-Ross's [39] work on the stages of grief remains a valuable guide to assisting those who are suffering from situational depression.)

The cumulative result of a series of losses, if the person is able to cope effectively with them, is the gradual weakening of the tendency toward attachment and the blossoming of a more universal love. The blossoming of a higher love that leads to emotional stability and self-fulfillment cannot happen overnight, however. This is a fundamental, painstaking developmental process in the human being. It is perhaps one of life's most important tasks.

Mental Illness

Mental illness occurs primarily as a result of ego imbalances. An insufficiently developed ego is as harmful as an overly developed one. The ego is the mental mechanism that creates the sense of separation among individuals. A weak ego, or a poorly differentiated self, can result in schizophrenia. An ego that is oversized may result in delusions or depression.

Western psychology assigns the ego a central role in its definition of mental health. Ego development in childhood is rightly considered to be absolutely central to a healthy personality. But, in adulthood, after a basic sense of self-confidence is established, the ego actually can be a source of severe mental dysfunction and intense suffering. It is the ego that makes one feel that a certain goal must be accomplished. It is the ego that compares oneself to others. It is the ego that condemns others. In this arena, insights from Eastern spiritual traditions have much to offer Western psychology.

Alan Watts[40] introduced the Eastern concept of ego transcendence to modern Western psychology. But even before Watts, James[41] described the same experience: "It is but giving your little private convulsive self a rest, and finding that a greater Self is there." The ego—or *small self*—creates a sense of separation and distance. It is also the source of ambition, hope, and fear. Many Westerners actually believe that transcending the ego is something to be feared. It smells of personal destruction, or of insanity. The paradox is that, through going beyond oneself, one finds oneself connected with all, free to act creatively, and secure in one's larger identity. We will explore the therapeutic power of ego transcendence further in Chapter 5.

Spiritual Illness

Spiritual pain is the most intense suffering of which humans are capable. We need only read the chronicles of the Christian saint John of the Cross or of the Indian saint Sri Ramakrishna to grasp the depths of pain experienced by a tortured soul. A person in spiritual distress is profoundly hopeless, sees no meaning in life or in death, and has no sense of connection with the world. He or she has a total alienation and sense of the worthlessness of life. Spiritual distress is a hallmark of modern life. The existentialist writers describe it with artistry, but the picture itself is harsh.

Depression and suicide are symptoms of spiritual despair. The rate of suicide is highest in industrialized societies. Even more common are the problems of cancer and heart disease. It is now apparent that these major killers of industrialized humanity are connected with spiritual distress, for such distress can lead to significant impairments in immunity. We can also infer this from the large body of research that indicates the health and recovery-promoting benefits of optimism, social support, and prayer.[42,43] A recent study indicated that elderly persons with a subjective feeling of spiritual support attribute their sense of health and well-being to this support.

Lack of faith is a fundamental characteristic of spiritual despair. One need not have belief in a personal God in order to have faith. One does need, however, a basic sense of trust that life is good overall and can bring one satisfaction and joy. Pessimism is a sign of spiritual distress. A lack of humor is another sign of spiritual distress.

Many share the opinion that the problem of substance abuse in industrialized society is largely due to the spiritual illness of its population. A lack of meaning and purpose in life, the loss of family and other strong and enduring social ties, and an impoverished materialist culture foster the alienation and hopelessness of a people. Beyond suicide and depression as obvious sequelae, we may consider the high rate of cancer in these societies as also being related, in part, to the impaired immune function that accompanies such a state of consciousness. The key to the preventive care and healing of a sick society lies in restoring a basic spiritual health to its members.

ILLNESS AS A CLEANSING

In many traditions, illness is looked upon as a cleansing of body, mind, or spirit. This is such a widespread belief that it deserves consideration. After a severe illness of even short duration, a person is weak and delicate. He or she is also much more sensitive to inner and outer sensations and vibrations. Sound, light, smell, taste, touch—all of one's senses—are heightened. Florence Nightingale[44] was very astute in her observations of this delicate condition of the sick. Why is this so? Because the sick have been cleansed. Their senses have been fine-tuned. Cleansing makes an instrument more sensitive, less clouded. People also appear different after extreme sickness. Their skin seems translucent and shining. Their eyes are bright. Their features are refined. There is an aura of light and an inner clarity. A process of purification has occurred.

Many of the symptoms that accompany illness are methods the body uses to clean itself. Diarrhea, vomiting, fever, sweating, and discharge all serve this purpose. Disease-causing elements such as microbes, foreign bodies, and pollutants are being eliminated.

Emotional and mental illness can also be viewed as cleansing processes. The same principles are operating. Expressing negative or harmful emotions or thoughts is the first step toward gaining control over and eventually eliminating them. The process of release may appear to be a mental illness. Certain psychotherapies are based on this principle. For example, primal therapy encourages clients to express primitive, basic emotions such as rage, competitiveness, or grief in as direct a manner as possible in order to purge themselves. Primal therapists believe that only then can one develop positive emotions and thought patterns.

From the evolutionary viewpoint, deep-seated or primitive emotions should neither be suppressed nor deliberately brought to the surface. The best way to further one's growth is to try to neutrally observe the workings of one's mind without identifying with its thoughts or feelings. Mental processes and products are not the expression of one's true self. They are like waves on a deep ocean of the infinite self, that aspect of the person that is eternal and unchanging. Thoughts and feelings come and go and cannot be relied upon to reveal the truth of things.

When one views illness as a cleansing process, the approach to healing is quite different from that of mainstream medicine. There is a fundamental confidence in the body's ability to heal itself through the cleansing symptoms. Unless the symptoms are so severe as to threaten life, the approach will be to not interfere with the pathological process. Naturopathic medicine and homeopathy are actually designed to work synergistically with the symptoms of illness.

The belief that illness is an expression of the body's effort to cleanse itself is consistent with the evolutionary paradigm of this book. Cleansing will allow higher frequency vibrations to resonate in the system. Through cleansing, we can increase our sensitivity to universal and higher consciousness. Perhaps this is why people who suffer a major illness often develop an aura of dignity and wisdom.

CONCLUSION

Illness can occur at any level of consciousness. The higher the level from which the problem arises, the more difficult it is to heal. Likewise, healing at the highest level possible will be the most effective approach. Illness usually is a reflection of an imbalance among the various levels of consciousness, although some illnesses may be purely due to karma.

Thus, illness brings a message well worth heeding. It is an indicator of maladjustment. From the evolutionary viewpoint, the solution to one's health problems lies in learning the lessons that illness brings. Once these are learned, the disease or illness will no longer be necessary. If physical pathology is extensive, a disease may not be reversible, but if a profound transformation has occurred, the disease will be considered a valued and respected teacher.

Although modern medicine treats disease, it does not treat illness. It tries to find a disease for every illness. A patient goes to the doctor complaining of not feeling well. The doctor orders numerous diagnostic tests. When the results all come back negative (which really means positive, from the patient's point of view), the doctor says, "There is nothing wrong with you. You are very healthy." The patient leaves feeling dissatisfied, for she knows that she is not well. She is ill, even though she has no disease. Treating illness is the real challenge for a healer. We will discuss ways of approaching the healing of illness in Chapter 5.

CHAPTER 4

DEATH

The subject of death is of utmost importance in human life, since humans know they will eventually die. Voltaire attributed this knowledge to experience; Heidegger considered it to be an immanent, a priori concept in human consciousness. Regardless of why we possess this awareness, the fact that we do possess it has profound consequences. One may say that the awareness of death permeates the entire civilization.

Health professionals, in particular, must come to terms with the issue of death. It is interesting to observe that, in most medical and nursing schools, the subject of death is minimally addressed in the curriculum. It may seem that to acknowledge the inevitability of death is to challenge the raison d'être of medicine. Yet the only thing we can be absolutely sure of is that we will die. What has this to say of health care providers, when most people spend their entire life in denial of this truth? We act as if we are immortal, engaging in behaviors that clearly may lead to death. We also treat others as if they will always be with us, not recognizing how precious and fragile each life really is.

Why is the only species that is aware of its own mortality so intent on denying it? It would make sense that awareness of death serves some evolutionary purpose, or it would not have emerged in the course of evolution. Suppressing this awareness is an affront to human evolution. Modern Western cultures are worse than many others at acknowledging the reality of death. They have few traditions or rituals to help with the actual experience of dying. It is the norm for death to occur in a hospital, where the patient is often alone—at best, in the presence of detached health care providers. In the evolutionary paradigm, awareness of one's personal mortality is an important step in the evolution of consciousness. Only by cultivating the art of dying can we practice the art of living. The great philosopher Spinoza[45] wrote, "A free man thinks of nothing less than of death, and his wisdom is not a meditation upon death but a meditation upon life." (Prop LXVII).

THE NATURE OF DEATH

In the framework of evolutionary healing, our perspective on death is based upon the ancient teaching of the Upanishads, expressed most beautifully in the *Bhagavad Gita*.[46] In this excerpt from the much larger epic called *Mahabharata*, a dialogue between the Lord (incarnate in human form) and the great warrior Arjuna takes place. Arjuna is hesitating at the beginning of an historic battle in which he will be forced to engage in mortal combat with his own relatives over an issue of crucial moral significance. Arjuna does not want to kill his relatives. To help him accept his duty as a righteous warrior, the Lord (in the form of Krishna) explains to him the true nature of death.

Krishna explains that, in fact, no one dies or is born. It is only the body that dies and is born. The real person, the soul, never dies. It is never born. It is immortal, and nothing can destroy it. The soul takes on one body after another. "As a man discarding worn-out clothes, takes other new ones, likewise the embodied soul, casting off worn-out bodies, enters into others which are new"[46] (II,22). Therefore, there is no reason to grieve or fear the death of oneself or of others.

We demonstrated in Chapter 1 that reincarnation explains more of the facts of life than does any other view and how it has been well documented through the research of Dr. Ian Stevenson. This is a subject on which health professionals usually remain silent, believing perhaps that it is unprofessional to offer an opinion. There is ample evidence to support the theory of reincarnation, and it is a widely held belief around the world. Socrates, the father of Western philosophy, advocated this view[47]. In fact, reincarnation was part of official Catholic doctrine until it was suppressed at the Second Council of Constantinople in 553. There is ample justification for discussing at least the possibility of reincarnation with those patients who express an interest in the subject. It may provide substantial therapeutic benefit.

It is helpful to examine why many people have an intense fear of death. One of the most common fears related to death is of the pain that may be associated with dying. There is also fear of personal extinction. There may be fear of the unknown, of what happens after death. If we do not believe that we cease to exist after death, we still do not know exactly what to expect in our new circumstances. For those who believe in hell, there is an added worry. It would be helpful if we could know what death and any possible existence after death actually involve. But our dilemma is this: How can we know about death? Those who die are the only ones who really know. Is there a way of understanding these mysteries?

Strangely, we do have access to some reports of what happens after death. In the past 20 years there has been a substantial body of research published on people who have had near-death experiences, which are actually after-death experiences. Dr. Raymond Moody[48,49] is the pioneer in this field, but his findings have now been replicated in other countries and by other researchers.[50,51]

There is a remarkable similarity in the stories told by survivors of death. All of these survivors maintain that they felt no pain at the time of their death. They were outside their bodies, observing with a peculiar detachment what was happening to them in the minutes after their death. They report a sense of great peace, although there is feeling for those left behind. (This feeling may be so strong that it pulls the person back to life.) There is a realization that consciousness continues after death. There is usually the sensation of moving at great speed, often through a tunnel. There is no fear associated with this journey. There is the sense of being watched over, as well as the sense that a loving presence is waiting at the end of the tunnel. Those who have had a near-death experience describe a presence manifesting complete unconditional love in the afterdeath realm.

Physicians and neurological researchers have proposed many theories in an effort to explain the near-death experience as a series of electrochemical events in the brain. All fall short of the task. British neurologist Peter Fenwick[51] examines the common physiological and psychological hypotheses that attempt to explain near-death experiences. He concludes that "either science is missing a fundamental link which would explain how organized experiences can arise in a disorganized brain, or that some forms of experience are transpersonal—that is, they depend on a mind which is not inextricably bound up with a brain" (p. 236).

The most compelling evidence that there is an actual consciousness that remains outside of the body after death is found in near-death survivors' descriptions of places and events that were not physically accessible to them. For example, the roof of the hospital is described in detail, or a conversation that took place in a remote part of the building or city is repeated. Observations such as these are a common part of the near-death experience. The only feasible explanation is that personal consciousness survives death and it is not constrained by space or time.

Dr. Moody notes a remarkable correspondence between the early stages of death described by the ancient classic, *The Tibetan Book of the Dead*[52], and his subjects' accounts of near-death experiences. Borman[53] summarizes the similarities:

> Moody recounts the same radical change in consciousness, including finding itself outside of the physical body, watching the preparation for the funeral just as his subjects watched the attempts at resuscitation of the body; the confusion and self-questioning of the dead person about his present state as being in fact death; regret; depression; lingering near familiar artifacts, people, and places; possession of a strange new non-material and "shining" body; ability to penetrate solid walls and rocks without resistance; instantaneous travel; new dimensions and clarity of thought and perception; great lucidity and keenness; meeting

other similar beings; meeting a clear pure light; feeling deep peace, contentment; and the review, as if on film, of one's entire life, not judgmentally, but with feelings of loving acceptance and of interest to learn the lessons that life experience offers, with no lying to oneself or to the being of light, possible (p. 69).

The Tibetan Book of the Dead deserves respectful study by anyone who has a serious interest in the subject of death. It provides a unique contribution to humanity's knowledge in this area. Read at the bedside of the dying and also to the deceased after the time of death, it provides guidance as the spirit moves into the postdeath realms. One of the most significant insights of this scripture is that each person's afterdeath experiences are entirely dependent upon his or her own mental content at the time of death. The afterdeath state is very similar to the dream state. In fact, for a time the deceased does not realize that he or she is dead and is experiencing sensations through a subtle body, much as sensations are experienced in a dream.

We have access also to insights into the nature of death from the writings and teachings of sages and mystics throughout the centuries. They have extraordinary abilities to grasp the hidden dimensions of reality. Ramananda[3] explains that death is a time of assimilation of experience and then of rest. Consciousness widens. The spirit learns the lessons of its past life. For the further development of the spirit, death is utterly necessary. After some time (when measured in human terms), the soul takes on another mental, emotional, and physical body.

This is a sober and realistic explanation of what happens after dying. It promises neither heaven nor hell for the ordinary person who still has much growth to accomplish. Our consciousness after death does not really change drastically; it only becomes more itself as the attachments and distractions of earthly existence are left behind. Heaven may be the period of rest and rejuvenation in the higher and wider consciousness of death. Hell may be the period of life review that takes place soon after death, when the spirit understands the harm it has caused others and how different actions could have had better outcomes.

Emotional or mental suffering may occur for some time after death, as the person does not shed all of the layers of consciousness immediately. For example, a person who has committed suicide may suffer intense remorse as he or she realizes the irreversibility of his or her action. Or a person with excessive attachment will suffer from separation from the beloved. In such a case, he or she may be reborn soon and will eventually make contact again with his or her loved one.

WITNESSING DEATH

I have been with many people as they have died. It does not appear that this is a time of suffering. There may be some suffering prior to the actual death, though we certainly have enough knowledge and ability to make this very preventable. But, at a certain point, the person clearly moves into a different consciousness. We usually call it *unconscious*, but it is an awareness of a different order—one that is not visible to the outside observer. Consciousness appears to shift so that it is no longer focusing on the body or the physical surroundings, or even on the emotional surroundings of friends and family. The person begins to move on. This occurs before the actual moment of death, unless the death is sudden and unexpected. There is a tangible change in the air.

The person starts to depart, but for some time certain aspects of his or her consciousness linger. The length of this lingering varies a great deal. It seems to depend on whether the deceased is really ready to let go, or whether the loved ones left behind are ready to let go.

The friends and family who are left behind after the death of a loved one suffer intensely. Mourning is one of the deepest of human emotions. Death is as necessary for the evolution of those who are left behind as it is for those who depart. It shifts responsibility to new shoulders. It comes as a challenge for inner and outer adjustment, and it opens up new experience to the bereaved. It brings people together, helping them to understand how vulnerable we all really are. It softens hearts that are hard, and strengthens hearts that are weak. Our grief makes us intensely aware of our attachments and may inspire us to a more universal sympathy and love.

We often question the necessity of death at all. We object to the fact that all living things must die. Why is the universe so organized that death follows life as night follows day? The evolutionary journey is very complex, passing through countless stages and experiences of all sorts. If we accept the premise that we are units of evolving consciousness, we must accept the need for death. We could not possibly gather enough experience in one body to graduate from the school of life. We have a fairly good idea of what we need to accomplish, and we must be ready to keep coming back until we get it right. We mind death, but we don't question birth. Where has this baby come from? Who is he?

THE ART OF DYING

In order to grow in consciousness while dying, we must face death honestly. Denial serves no purpose in this process. First, in order to face death honestly, it helps to realize that life itself is nothing but a terminal illness. Its end is certain. When one's death appears imminent, the opportunity for great strides in personal evolution exists. A radical transformation is possible.

Talking openly about the reality of one's situation with family and friends is important. This is not always so easy, however. Family and friends may not want to deal with the emotions that are aroused. A sympathetic nurse or other health professional may be more comfortable in discussing such issues. Talking openly with someone will help to identify whatever fears and concerns are present.

It also is important to clarify one's thoughts or beliefs about existence after death. Health care providers should be careful not to make assumptions about a person's true beliefs based on his or her professed religious affiliation. Every individual forms very personal views about death, despite what he or she may be taught in church. The subject should be respectfully raised, with a readiness to discuss various points of view. For this, reading from the world's various spiritual traditions can be of value. We mentioned earlier some excellent resources from Eastern traditions. Plato's reports of Socrates' conversations and teachings are a rich source of insight as well.

Some form of meditation, or centering prayer, will facilitate one's journey of self-exploration and self-healing. Meditation helps the dying person make contact with that aspect of his or her inner self, which endures beyond death. Chapter 2 described the impact of meditation on conscious energy, and Chapter 5 will describe this practice in greater detail.

Music that calms and lifts the spirit can also help the individual become get centered and focused. It is also an effective means of pain relief[54]. Self-exploration and expression through keeping a journal, writing poetry, or doing other artistic activities will facilitate one's passage.

At the same time that one is anticipating and preparing for death, it is also helpful to continue with normal life activities as much as possible. Every experience will have an intensity and poignancy that never existed before. The dying person looks at the world with a unique perspective, and this contributes greatly to the evolution of his or her consciousness. Often, people who are dying report that they recognize the value and worth of all life, feel a heightened sensory pleasure in everyday experience, and may even perceive a special luminosity in people and objects.

It is extremely important that the person who is anticipating imminent death be encouraged to reconcile his or her relationships, bringing as much honesty and forgiveness into them as possible. This will provide greater peace of mind as death is encountered, and it will help in the postmortem journey of consciousness. A tortured consciousness will have difficulty moving on. Such a consciousness may have to return quickly into a physical body and into circumstances similar to the current life. This is an area where effective counseling and support can be helpful.

Conscious dying requires that one be physically comfortable in order to free one's energy and attention. Effective pain management is crucial. Pain management does not imply sedation. Many people are resistant to using narcotics because they do not want to lose their mental faculties. They believe— incorrectly—that morphine or other narcotics will cause severe drowsiness. This happens only initially. As the body is freed from the grip of pain, it relaxes dramatically, and sleep is a natural reaction. Morphine also has a direct nervous system depressant effect, but only for the first few days of use. Then the brain becomes tolerant of this effect, and relatively normal wakefulness is then possible. Experts in pain management also know how to combine narcotics with other, nonnarcotic drugs and devices in order to be able to minimize the requirement for morphine.

Other discomforts associated with terminal illness may include nausea, loss of function of body parts, incontinence, and so on. In our age, we have excellent measures available to mitigate all such discomforts. Referral to a hospice program can be extremely beneficial. Hospice professionals are very skilled at helping create an environment—at home whenever possible—that is conducive to the patient's maximum functioning and comfort.

If it is possible to anticipate the time of death, it will be important for family and close friends to gather so that they can say good-bye openly and give the dying permission to depart. It is common nursing wisdom, based on millions of hours of attending at deaths, that patients whose families give permission for their departure die peacefully and easily. This can be explained to the family, as it may be the last gift that they give to their beloved.

We are all on the verge of death every moment. We should cultivate this awareness, not push it away. It will make us more selective about what we do with our time and with whom we spend it. It will make us all enjoy the ordinary activities of life with an extraordinary appreciation.

CONCLUSION

Dying is simply the body's winding down. Observe how an animal with a serious illness behaves. This will teach an important lesson about how to live well while dying. An animal has no awareness that its life is ending. Without that awareness, it does not make much of its disease or pain. It simply carries on, focusing its attention on its usual habits and routines. Animals do not suffer; they simply feel pain and deal with it.

Of course, we can never and should never revert back to animal consciousness, but it is instructive to observe how much of human suffering comes from mental and emotional responses. As humans, we can make our awareness of mortality a powerful transformative experience. Both the dying and the surviving can find depths of meaning and the opportunity for accelerated evolution of consciousness.

Why must humans suffer? Because suffering spurs one on in the growth of consciousness. Suffering in this sense is necessary for spiritual growth. However, its purpose is to give one the opportunity to rise above it, to get to a place beyond the mind and emotions, a place where there is a lasting peace and maybe even a taste of joy. Dying need not to be a time of suffering. It can be a time of tremendous clarity and calm. It can bring insights and wisdom that no amount of pleasurable living can provide. It deepens consciousness, paving the way for one's next step forward.

Chapter 5

Healing

A New View of Healing

It is important to understand the role that disease and illness play in human evolution. At the animal or plant level, disease seems rather straightforward. It is due to organic or physical dysfunction. The stronger members of the species survive, whereas the weak succumb. But in the human species, desires, ego, and attachments enter the picture. Disease no longer serves to eliminate the weak. We launch an aggressive fight against disease.

When a person asks to be healed, she means she wants a cure. She thinks that her problem is physical, and the only thing she knows is physical healing. But from an evolutionary viewpoint healing has more to do with heart, mind, and spirit than with the body. The body is a consciousness just like those other dimensions, and the most effective healing takes place in the highest possible level of conscious energy. Healing takes place when, as a result of the evolution of consciousness, a greater harmony and integration of the various levels of consciousness occur.

The word *heal* comes from the Old English word for *whole*. How does a human being become more whole? He or she becomes more integrated and harmonious in purpose and function. The various levels of consciousness in an ordinary person have different goals and processes. In the average person, there is significant conflict among them. If our levels of consciousness could argue, the conversation might go something like this:

Body: Hey, all I want is a little comfort. I need a warm home, a soft bed, lots of sleep, and food that pleases my tongue and stomach. I need sexual pleasure whenever the urge arises. I prefer strong sensations to mild ones. I only feel alive when my senses are fully engaged. It feels so good!

Heart: You are disgusting. I am asking you to commit yourself to love and cherish at least one other person in the world besides yourself. I need to live on something more than physical comfort. I need to see and hear and read beautiful, artistic creations. In fact, I need to produce something beautiful myself. I crave the joy of loving a spouse and a child. I want somebody to love me exclusively, to love no one else as much as they love me. I need to go outside of myself and experience the beauty of nature. I need to feel needed by others and to feel that I am a good person.

Mind: You both are very primitive. I need to control you or you will interfere with my ability to see the world calmly and clearly. Logic and rational thought can solve all the problems that you both create. Emotion is unreliable, and the body should be controlled so that it is my instrument. We should be very careful about basing our lives on untestable concepts like love and God. Art is fine as far as it goes, but mostly it is just a waste of time. I think we should spend more time studying philosophy and history. You two need to be controlled or you will destroy the world.

Spirit: You all are living an illusion. Don't you know that only the spirit is real? Everything else is going to die. Why should you put so much energy into anything that will not last forever? The best thing you can do with your time is to think of eternity and divinity, and to prepare for your death. God is not a person who made you and then forgot about you. God is in you, and you are in God. It really is a waste to build all these relationships that are going to end in a few decades (at the most) anyway. And to think that the body is the main source of joy is sheer stupidity.

No wonder many people feel inner turmoil most of the time! These are very strong, conflicting forces inside the individual. As we discussed earlier, poor health often results from such inner conflicts. Healing, then, moves the person from a state of inner conflict and disharmony into one of greater integration and unity. Unity is possible when all aspects of the individual are geared toward the same goal. The individual will determine his or her main goal. It may be to creatively express oneself through art, to serve others through one's profession, to excel in sports or in business, or simply to create a loving family for one's children. For some, it may be to cultivate one's spiritual core. Whatever one's life goals, health means that all the aspects of one's being are working together to support one's goals.

As we showed earlier, the subtler, higher frequencies of conscious energy are more powerful than the lower frequencies. This holds the key to true healing. Whatever problem exists, we must find its cure in the higher layers of our being. Low back pain, for example, often appears to be due to a physical injury or trauma. However, it has become increasingly apparent to rehabilitation experts that the cause of many cases of chronic back pain is in mental processes that suppress unconscious emotions. Dr. John Sarno[55] has been a pioneering researcher in this area. Even diseases that create profound pathological alterations, such as cancer or heart disease, are susceptible to influence by mental and spiritual factors.

How do the higher orders of consciousness modulate the lower so that healing can take place? As explained in Chapter 1, the higher levels of consciousness have a greater capacity to create change (i.e., to use the will) than do the lower levels. The same is true of the capacity for self-modification (i.e., changing one's emotions or affection). The higher levels are capable of modulating the levels below through sympathetic vibrations.

A troubled and turbulent emotional consciousness, therefore, will in turn cause alterations in organic energy, leading to dysfunction of the neuroendocrine and immune systems. The person will then be susceptible to diseases such as cancer, autoimmune illness, and so on. Illness at the mental or spiritual level will have similar effects. Seasoned clinicians have always recognized the profound influence that mind and spirit have on health and illness. We now have an overwhelming body of research that confirms this clinical wisdom.

MECHANISMS AND LAWS OF EVOLUTION APPLIED TO THE HEALING PROCESS

Our view is that healing is an evolutionary process. It will be important, therefore, to apply the mechanisms and principles of evolution we outlined in Chapter 1 to the healing process.

Reincarnation

As we noted earlier, the soul requires a vast range of experience for its evolution. Reincarnation gives the soul access to many different personalities, occupations, cultures, and ages. Eventually, these experiences provide us with true wisdom and a glimmer of love. The hard knocks of life facilitate great strides in the evolution of consciousness. Pain and other physical experiences (paralysis, seizures, dysfunction, etc.) that come with disease can create a very deep impression in an otherwise insensitive consciousness. They deliver their message very effectively. The message may not be apparent while the individual is enduring the disease, but insight may come after recovery, or the soul assimilates it after death.

This means that we should not make relief of suffering the primary goal of our healing efforts. The physical, emotional, mental, and spiritual pain associated with disease has an evolutionary purpose. The person who has been diagnosed with a terminal disease, for example, should be encouraged to express rather than suppress the fears, sense of loss, and spiritual distress he or she is experiencing. In a supportive atmosphere, this will be of more value than providing a tranquilizer to dull the experience. We discussed in Chapter 4 the importance of alleviating physical pain, but this is not the main task of healing.

Karma

Reincarnation and the law of karma are, of course, directly related. Karma is action, and every action creates a reaction. Karmic reactions extend across the span of many lifetimes. As we participate in healing, we need to recognize that the law of karma will determine the ultimate outcome.

But the law of karma can also be harnessed to great effectiveness in the healing process. The direct impact of new action may be of enormous benefit. One can control new actions and create new karmas. One can choose to exercise regularly, to eat healthy foods, to resolve troubled relationships, and to transform negative feelings and thoughts. All such efforts will bear fruit through the same law of karma that brings disease. There is always the opportunity to prevent or modify disease by self-effort.

The Laws of Evolution

Law of Necessity.   Every experience comes out of evolutionary necessity. It has a role to play in one's growth. Recognizing this is a crucial step in the healing process. The wise patient will embrace the challenge presented by disease and illness.

Understanding that illness comes for a reason does not preclude the effort to heal. One can try to understand the message and to learn from it. Self-effort is crucial in evolutionary healing. One may then grow in knowledge, feeling, and will through illness and suffering.

Law of Integration.   The law of integration explains that the development of each level of consciousness is subordinate to the integrity and evolution of the person as a whole. No single level of consciousness has an independent existence. The chemical behavior of molecules is constrained by the organizing power of organic energy. For example, an iron atom in a hemoglobin molecule does not have the same magnetic properties as elemental iron. In turn, the physiological needs of the organism bow to the influence of mind and spirit. A mother may sacrifice her own life to save her child. A scholar working on a difficult problem may not leave his office for days or weeks. He will neglect food, exercise, and sleep.

Overall, the state of health of the human species is poorer than that of animals. Chronic diseases increase in frequency as civilization advances. We pay the price of our evolution in the coin of disease. This does not mean that we must resign ourselves to the inevitability of ill health. Ultimately, as all aspects of the person become integrated and balanced, high-level health will emerge.

Law of Sacrifice.   The law of sacrifice complements the law of integration. One may choose to sacrifice certain desires of organic energy in order to develop subtler levels of consciousness. Nutritious food, adequate rest, and regular exercise are the needs of organic energy and form the foundation of good health. Even these at times may be sacrificed, only temporarily, for the sake of developing one's higher levels of consciousness.

Ultimately, fulfillment of higher level needs has a trickle-down effect. An actual transformation at the lower levels takes place, so that old cravings and needs change; suppression can be harmful to the organism. The *law of sacrifice* refers to a natural refinement and purification in all levels of consciousness that takes place in the course of evolution. It does not advocate artificial, externally imposed repression of natural instincts and needs.

Law of Compressed Processes.   The law of compressed processes is particularly relevant to the process of healing. It explains that the pace of evolution is always increasing. Every action leaves an imprint that makes reproduction of the action easier the next time it is attempted. When one attempts to change habits into a healthier pattern, this law becomes relevant. Every time a new behavior is performed, it becomes easier to reproduce. The less often an unhealthy behavior is enacted, the easier it is to eradicate. The body itself has a habit of illness or of health that can be changed with effort.

HEALING THERAPIES AT VARIOUS LEVELS OF CONSCIOUSNESS

Even if one is not afflicted with an illness, there is always the possibility of being healthier. The alternative health movement has gained wide popularity because of this understanding. Perfect health is sold in the marketplace. Wellness centers are proliferating as do pizza stands. Although an extraordinary person can become perfectly healthy, there are many general measures that everyone can take to improve health. We discussed many of these in Chapter 2.

In this chapter, we set forth a scheme for classifying the hundreds of healing therapies available. Our system is based on the levels of conscious energy that have been discussed throughout this book. Because all dimensions are in constant interaction, a given therapy affects every level. However, it is useful to place each therapy within the level that it affects most directly. The result is a typology of therapeutic measures that can facilitate a rational and comprehensive approach to healing.

Physical Healing

Cleansing the body.   We discussed the idea of physical cleansing in Chapter 3. We now will explore the measures that can be taken to accomplish it. In naturopathic medicine, cleansing is a key concept. In the normal processes of life, waste products are generated. These waste products can accumulate and interfere with optimal cellular, tissue, or organ functioning.

Eliminating free radical buildup.   Free radicals are perhaps the best known of toxic metabolic by-products. When body cells are exposed to a high level of pollutants, as when a person lives in an urban area, they generate excessive amounts of free radicals that, in turn, can cause serious damage to the body.

Heart disease and cancer are directly related to the accumulation of free radicals. They are the top two killers of American adults. Researchers are searching intensively for substances that help to counteract the buildup of free radicals in the body. Because the chemical process called *oxidation* generates free radicals, many antioxidants have been researched and demonstrated to have preventive effects in terms of both heart disease and cancer.

Antioxidants are available in a variety of forms. Vitamins C, E, and beta-carotene are the major antioxidant vitamins. Nutritional supplements derived from certain fruits, such as grape seed and tamarind, contain antioxidants hundreds of times more potent than these vitamins. Green tea and black tea are also excellent sources of antioxidants.

Dietary measures to cleanse the body.   Fasting and increasing water intake are the best-known methods of physical cleansing. The theory underlying these practices is, again, related to the fact that metabolism of food results in the generation of waste products that must be eliminated so that they will not harm the system. Occasionally reducing or eliminating food intake allows the body to clear out accumulated waste. A liberal intake of water during a fast and at other times is crucial, for this helps waste to be circulated to the kidneys and excreted in the urine. A weekly one-day or monthly weekend fast can be very helpful.

True fasting means having no caloric intake whatsoever. But a juice diet for a short period of time can also help the body to rest and be cleansed. The *juice fast* consists of simple carbohydrates. These are the easiest nutrients for the body to assimilate and metabolize. Proteins and fats generate much larger waste molecules that are more complex to eliminate. A cleansing diet should be a short-term change from the usual balanced diet. It is difficult to maintain one's strength on a prolonged cleansing diet.

Hydrotherapy.   The therapeutic use of water, this is one of the most ancient methods of healing. Baths are a common form of hydrotherapy. Immersing the body in warm water increases the blood flow to the skin's surface, where it can release waste products through the pores. Thus, it helps clean more than dirt from the skin. Hot baths also raise body temperature and induce sweating, both of which can be helpful in fighting an acute infection. Bacteria and viruses are sensitive to heat, and sweating is another means of eliminating toxic wastes. Many people also find cold-water bathing to be an invigorating and health-promoting measure. Whereas a hot bath may weaken, a cold swim energizes.

Mud bathing and localized mud packs are another method of healing believed to draw waste products and toxins out through the skin. Mud can help stomach pain, joint pain, and headaches. It is cooling and astringent. It may also help draw out toxins from infections and tumors.

Cleansing the intestines.   Enemas are the most common method of cleaning the intestines. Many patients report that self-administered enemas relieve headaches, stomachaches, and other minor ailments. Colon hydrotherapy is a technique of total intestinal cleansing. The large intestine's main function is to process and eliminate the waste products of food digestion and absorption. Largely because of the modern diet's insufficient fiber content, much of the waste, unfortunately, remains in the walls of the large intestine.

Colon therapists maintain that this stagnating waste produces toxic substances that contribute to many chronic health problems, including fatigue, headaches, premenstrual syndrome, irritable bowel syndrome, and—even more seriously—to life-threatening problems like colon cancer and inflammatory bowel disease.

Natural medicine practitioners make much of the harmful effects of toxins. They explain that these toxins, when they are mobilized and eliminated from the body, create a response in the body called a *healing crisis*. During the crisis, the person may experience headache, fatigue, nausea, or vomiting. Naturopaths maintain that this is an important step in the cleansing process. If the toxins are not stirred up, they cannot be eliminated. In the long run, they do much more harm if they are left alone to quietly accumulate.

We can turn to chaos theory, as explained in Chapter 1, to help explain the healing crisis. During a period of disequilibrium, rapid change to a higher degree of organization is possible. The healing crisis is one such time of disequilibrium. New patterns, or higher levels, of health become possible. There are thousands of anecdotal reports in the literature of spontaneous healing that has been apparently induced by methods of physical cleansing.

We can also appreciate the value of cleansing when we remember that the body is made of conscious energy vibrating at various frequencies. In Chapter 3, we noted that higher frequency vibrations are more powerful and represent a more subtle and refined consciousness than do lower frequencies. Cleansing the body allows its energy to vibrate at a higher frequency. It is more sensitive to higher frequency vibrations from both within and without. Emotional, mental, and spiritual energies resonate freely in a purified body. This is why, in all spiritual traditions, fasting and other cleansing measures are valued.

Strengthening the Body. A strong body can support the flights of heart, mind, and spirit. A weak body can affect one's mood and attitudes, and it tends to foster pessimism. One of the indicators of good health is a reserve of strength and energy to meet unexpected demands.

Exercise. Exercise is an important means of strengthening the body. One must use the muscles in order to maintain their strength. This is a physiological law. As a starting point for couch potatoes, the rule is that any form of activity is better than inactivity. The natural tendency as one ages is to become more sedentary. Resisting one's natural inertia is an important step toward healing.

If we look at sufferers of arthritis, we can see how important it is to keep moving. This chronic degenerative disease destroys the joints slowly but steadily. The individual who continues to maintain normal activity despite pain and stiffness will never give the joints the chance to stop functioning.

Even a few days of inactivity can make it much more difficult to return to the previous level of functioning.

Exercise can also contribute directly and powerfully to healing disease. Many studies have shown that exercise is effective in the treatment of depression[56]. In the treatment of Type II diabetes, exercise is absolutely central to maintaining control of blood glucose. Exercise makes the muscles more sensitive to insulin, helping them absorb and utilize glucose. There is a tribe of American Indians in New Mexico known as *The Walkers* who have an extraordinarily high incidence of Type II diabetes. Whereas normally the majority of them would be expected to require medication, none of the tribal members need it. They conduct all of their daily activities and commerce on foot, averaging at least 10 miles a day. All have excellent control of their diabetes.

Exercise also plays a major role in reducing the risk of heart disease. It does so by several mechanisms. First, aerobic exercise raises HDL cholesterol levels, and this protects against the development of coronary artery disease. Regular aerobic exercise also strengthens the heart, just as it does any other muscle, thereby allowing the heart to use less oxygen to do the same amount of work as an unfit heart muscle would use. Finally, exercise contributes to the relaxation and widening of the arteries, thereby reducing blood pressure and allowing greater blood flow to the heart and other organs. Weight-bearing exercise is an important measure to prevent osteoporosis.

Nutrition. Food also gives strength and energy to the body. It provides the building blocks for cells and tissues. Protein is necessary for building muscle tissue. Carbohydrates also are important, especially in providing a quick source of energy. Fats, though they take longer to be converted into energy, provide more calories per gram than either proteins or carbohydrates.

Nutrition plays a crucial role in healing. The field of nutritional medicine has evolved into a true scientific discipline. We now have *nutriceuticals*, foods that are transformed into medicinal agents for the treatment of specific diseases. An example is the use of defatted fenugreek seed to lower postprandial (postmeal) blood glucose levels. Omega-6 fatty acids raise HDL levels. Certain oils are used to control seizures.

Massage and Manual Therapies. Massage has a direct healing effect on the body. It improves circulation, stimulates lymph drainage, and can actually stimulate the immune response[57]. Even more important, it induces the relaxation response. Massage also serves as a powerful means of emotional healing. Touch is a fundamental human need; without it, neither children nor adults can thrive.

Techniques of manual manipulation include chiropractic and osteopathy. These systems of healing are based on the theory that structure determines function. They are particularly helpful in problems such as low back pain, neck pain, and headaches. The fact that these therapies involve touch also contributes to their effectiveness, no doubt.

Organic Healing

Healing at the organic level is even more effective than physical healing. We noted previously that organic energy is a higher order of consciousness and regulates the body's physical processes. If a disorder can be corrected at the organic level rather than at the physical level, a more long-lasting solution to the problem is found. There are several powerful therapies that specifically target the organic level of consciousness. They modulate the entire organism, not just a single part. Three major therapeutic systems modify organic energy: homeopathy, acupuncture, and Ayurveda. Therapeutic touch and botanical medicine are also measures that are believed to work at the organic level of energy.

Homeopathy.   Samuel Hahnemann[58] developed homeopathy in the early 19th century. He was a highly respected German physician who realized that the common medical practices of his day were crude and ineffective. He believed that the body has a defense mechanism that is self-regulating and self-healing. Hahnemann called it the *life force*, and he maintained that it regulates physiological processes. This belief correlates readily with our concept of organic consciousness.

When the body's defense mechanism becomes disordered, disease appears. The symptoms of a disease are actually the effort of the defense mechanism to regain equilibrium. Rather than suppressing or eliminating symptoms, then, healing must support the symptoms and allow them to do their work. Hahnemann experimented for decades with a wide variety of herbs and other medicinal agents. Realizing that symptoms must be supported rather than suppressed, he would first prove or test the potential medicine in healthy subjects and observe what the effects were. This would provide the clue to what diseases the given agents would be able to cure. Through his experimental observations, he developed the principle of *like cures like*.

What is important for us to understand is that this system of medical therapeutics is based on an understanding of the organic level of consciousness. Millions of people throughout the world rely on homeopathic practitioners for their main source of medical care. Homeopathy is a difficult system to test using the usual scientific method of double-blind, placebo-controlled clinical trials. Each person is treated individually, so that different homeopathic medicines will be prescribed for the same disease. There have, however, been several recent studies that support the effectiveness of homeopathic medicine for various health complaints.[59,60]

Acupuncture.   Acupuncture is one of the oldest known therapies. It falls within the larger system of traditional Chinese medicine. The *Nei Jing*, or *Yellow Emperor's Classic of Internal Medicine*[61], written in 206 B.C., describes the flow of vital energy along pathways in the body called *meridians*. These meridians correspond to different body organs, and the vital energy regulates their function. Again, we see that this therapy is based on a view that organic energy is a consciousness that regulates the physical body.

Traditional Chinese medicine further breaks down vital energy (*chi*) into two forces, yin and yang. These must remain in an optimal balance in order for health to exist. Insertion of needles into certain meridian points on the skin helps to keep these two forces in correct balance. This allows the entry and exit of internal as well as external yin and yang. The skin is the interface between cosmic energy and individual energy, and the meridians are the pathways for this energy.

Acupuncture has gained in acceptance by Western medicine to the point that there are now many managed care organizations and health insurers that offer or reimburse this treatment. It has been validated as an effective treatment for chronic and acute pain, anesthesia—even for major internal surgery—and a long list of health problems such as sinusitis, gastrointestinal dysfunction, and epilepsy.[62] Most Western practitioners try to explain its beneficial effects in pathophysiological terms. It is indeed true that the technique has profound pathophysiological effects. But this does not exclude the possibility that these effects are brought about by regulating the flow of vital energy.

Ayurveda.   *Ayurveda* is the Sanskrit word for *science of life*. This is the indigenous healing system of India, and it traces its roots back to nearly 1000 B.C. Ayurveda is a very sophisticated system that encompasses dietary, lifestyle, medicinal, herbal, spiritual, and surgical therapeutics.[63] In Ayurveda, the cosmos and the person, a microcosm, consist of three qualities (*satwa, rajas,* and *tamas*) and three *doshas,* humors (air, phlegm, and bile [*vat, kapha,* and *pitta*]). *Prana* is the life force and is responsible for organizing and regulating all the life processes. This concept is equivalent to our concept of organic energy.

A proper balance among the three qualities and humors is necessary for optimum health and to prevent disease. Each individual has a basic constitution, in which one of these three dominates, so that what is proper balance will vary from person to person. These qualities and humors can be adjusted by various lifestyle, medicinal, dietary, and environmental measures.

We see in all three of these healing traditions the primacy of organic energy. Each system has a long record of success. We must recognize the power of organic energy in any enlightened approach to medicine. It goes by various names—for example, *chi*, vital force, and *prana*—but it is the same basic energy that has been recognized and harnessed since the beginning of medicine.

Botanical Therapies.   Botanical therapies have properties that can be classified as both physical and organic. Herbs contain pharmacologically active substances that modulate the body's chemistry. In fact, many drugs are derived from plants. For example, taxol is a chemotherapeutic agent derived from a tree. Aspirin is derived from willow bark. The trend toward utilization of standardized herbal extracts in which the active ingredient is isolated and strengthened reflects the chemical view of herbs.

But there is another view that considers herbs to be therapeutic at the organic level of consciousness. From this perspective, it is the whole plant in its natural form that has properties that influence the organism as a whole. Therapeutically synergistic elements of the plant are found in the whole plant, and these are necessary for maximum healing benefit. Many herbalists believe that botanicals actually influence emotional and mental energies as well—indeed, some botanicals have been shown to do exactly this. St. John's Wort is an excellent herb for treating depression. Valerian is an excellent sleep aid.

Therapeutic Touch

Therapeutic touch is the intentional use of the hands to modulate the flow of organic energy. Close to 100,000 professionals in over 75 countries have been trained in this technique[64]. Therapeutic touch explicitly asserts that organic energy is the source of illness and healing.

Many studies have been conducted to test the efficacy of therapeutic touch. Overall, they suggest that this healing method can be of particular benefit in decreasing pain and anxiety and that it may be beneficial in enhancing wound healing.[65-68]

Emotional Healing

There is a field of emotional energy (traditionally called the *astral body*) comparable to the etheric body that encompasses organic energy. The astral body is responsible for the distinctive personality of each human being. It evolves in the course of one's lifetime with varying speed. Emotional healing is simply the acceleration of evolutionary development in the astral body. This development is from lower to higher emotions. Hatred, jealousy, lust, anger, greed, fear, and malevolence are lower emotions. We do not look upon them as sins, but as unhealthy patterns of response. Ramananda[2] explains that they generate poisons in the physical organism and damage the nervous system.

Emotional healing, then, is the transformation of negative emotions into positive emotions. Healing at the emotional level of consciousness is more challenging than is physical or organic healing. It requires lifelong effort, for many emotions are unconscious and deeply buried in one's personality. The first step in emotional healing is to bring one's patterns of emotional response into the light of conscious awareness. As discussed earlier, a person has certain automatic reactions based more on past experiences than on current reality. These reactions can color relationships and daily experience to such a degree that one becomes truly dysfunctional. A dramatic example of this is Post-Traumatic Stress Disorder.

There are many ways to achieve insight into one's emotional patterns. No matter what method is used—psychotherapy, keeping a diary, or group counseling—the effort can result in increased emotional health. From the evolutionary perspective, bringing emotional patterns into the light of consciousness subjects them to the more subtle, and therefore more powerful, energy of the rational mind. This can help to correct negative, self-destructive emotions. The conscious mind, however, cannot provide a final transformation of negative emotion into positive emotion. Moving from lust to love, from anger to tolerance, from greed to generosity—this evolution requires not only correct use of the rational mind, but also the transforming power of spiritual consciousness. The first step, however, is to expose one's emotional depths to the light of conscious awareness.

After one's emotional patterns are identified, it is helpful to find an outlet for expressing them constructively. Creative activities such as music, poetry, prose, and art are excellent outlets. A person without any outlet for emotional communication will encounter difficulty in achieving true health. (An example from current affairs is the vice president of the United States, Richard Cheney. This is an individual who, from all appearances, keeps all personal emotion tightly suppressed. One rarely sees a smile or any expression of feeling on his face. Though relatively young, he has suffered two heart attacks and had multiple-vessel bypass surgery while still in his forties.)

Social support provides an atmosphere in which emotional expression is encouraged and accepted, no matter what the content. It provides a state of emotional well-being that, in turn, allows a free flow of astral and organic energy with concomitant stimulation of the immune system. The positive effects on immune function associated with social support can increase the survival time of persons with cancer[42].

Recreation, relaxation, and play are also important vehicles for emotional healing. Partaking in the imaginative arts (e.g., cinema, fiction, and poetry) can provide opportunities for relief from unpleasant personal emotions and for vicarious expression of the range of human feelings. Inspiration to high emotions of love, courage, sacrifice, and the like also can be therapeutic and foster the evolution of consciousness.

One of the best vehicles for expanding the heart into higher emotions is service. Service to others provides a wonderful opportunity for emotional growth. This can take many forms, including taking care of animals. Indeed, pet therapy is now recognized to have substantial therapeutic benefit. Pets totally depend on humans for their life and well-being. In return they offer unconditional love. The healing power of service is an illustration of the larger principle that through giving we receive.

Mental Healing

Negative thoughts and attitudes are the source of untold misery and illness. Because of the power of the mind, negativity at this level has a profound impact on emotion, organic energy, and the body. It clearly interferes with the blossoming of the self. Often, negativity is directed towards oneself, and thoughts then become self-defeating. On the other hand, one can harness the power of the mind to great benefit in the healing process.

Mobilizing the Healing Power of the Mind.   Imagery can be an extremely effective way of using the conscious mind to stabilize troubled emotions and evoke the mind's self-healing powers. Imagery is the mental recall of specific sensations and images associated with a particular experience in an effort to facilitate relaxation, healing, or both. For example, after inducing relaxation by evoking an image of a relaxed and pleasant experience, one's conscious mind can be used to imagine the various components of the immune system attacking a tumor. Or one can visualize and invoke a spiritual force to enhance healing. Research suggests that imagery-relaxation may improve immune function[42]. Biofeedback and hypnosis are also effective measures that can focus the mind in ways that facilitate healing.

Values clarification is another tool for mental healing. Conflicting values can cause great mental suffering. One values family, but one also wants career success. If the two appear to be incompatible, a severe mental and emotional strain can result. One must examine all the competing values in one's life, prioritize them, decide what matters the most, and then plan one's time and activities accordingly. This can reduce much of the stress that accompanies complex modern life.

Graham[69] offers an interesting explanation of how the methods described contribute to healing. She explains that they modify the individual's relationship with, or experience of, time. One's sense of time, she asserts, is related to one's experience of stress, which is in turn related to many major diseases such as hypertension, heart disease, asthma, and diabetes. Prolonged stress reactions can also suppress the immune system.

Stress itself is a state of mental consciousness, particularly of the ego. The sense of *doership* is the fundamental source of human stress. One has the feeling of doing too much. Stress has extensive physiological effects that we know only too well. It is a crucial problem to resolve in the quest for healing. Stress results when one wishes not to be doing what one is doing or intensely desires a specific outcome that is beyond one's control. The ego is overinvested in results. One's identity and sense of self-esteem are at stake.

Here, then, lies the key to reducing stress. Either one should only do what one enjoys doing or one should attain a state in which one can enjoy anything. And one should be secure in one's self, no matter what the outcome. In practice, this is an enormously difficult state of mind to reach. But, little by little, one can make progress. The best way to resolve stress is to cultivate one's spiritual consciousness. The ego will then lose its grip on the personality. One can experience life's challenges and tasks, then, without anxiety or fear.

Music Therapy.   It is difficult to classify healing through music into a single level of consciousness. From our perspective, the level of influence of music depends not only on its source but also on the listener. Various types of music have their effect on different levels of consciousness. For example, rock music affects physical and organic consciousness because it originates from a consciousness that is operating from this base. On the other hand, Gregorian chant and classical Indian instrumental music originate from a strongly resonating spiritual consciousness and have a strong effect on the spiritual consciousness of the listener. Bach and Beethoven fall somewhere in between. The rich energy of music clearly has a strong healing potential[70].

Transcending the Ego. The first requirement of mental health is self-confidence. One can consider this requirement the need for a strong ego, but this is only true within certain limits. As discussed in Chapter 3, establishment of an intact ego is an important developmental task of childhood. But it is also true that, in the adult world, the ego is a source of much suffering when it pits one against the world.

Insights from Eastern spiritual traditions provide us with a way of resolving this dilemma. The ego creates a sense of separation from the world and others. Rather than crushing the ego, or dissolving it, which leads to psychosis, it is possible to transcend the ego, to cultivate the understanding that the boundary between self and others is illusory. It may be a boundary necessary for daily functioning, but it is an arbitrary and fluid boundary at best. When the ego is transcended, conflict dissolves. Stress disappears. Paradoxically, one becomes more free to find and express one's true self. Identifying with the self of all is a healing step that flows from one's spiritual center. We will discuss ways to arrive at this consciousness in the next section.

Spiritual Healing

Spiritual healing does not mean healing the spirit, for the spirit is perfect. It is always whole and healthy. *Spiritual healing* means simply allowing one's spirit to blossom and assume its rightful place in one's life. It is a priori the most effective way of healing, for spiritual consciousness is the highest frequency energy and can orchestrate all other conscious energies into harmony with its own vibration. The goal of spiritual healing, then, is to put oneself in tune with one's inner self, which means to be in tune with the infinite.

Meditation, prayer, and other means of connecting with the spirit are among the most ancient forms of healing known. Even in a culture in which one does not believe that evil spirits cause disease and good spirits cure, there is still ample justification for invoking spiritual consciousness to facilitate healing. Meditation is the most effective method of connecting with one's spiritual core and source. We have already addressed the methodology of meditation in Chapter 2.

It is important to clarify that our perspective on meditation is not biomedical. We do not consider its goal to be to induce relaxation, although this is clearly a positive side effect of meditation. For evolutionary healing, the value of meditation is in its ability to invoke high-frequency cosmic or divine consciousness, thereby transforming the meditator's consciousness as it begins to resonate with the higher frequencies. The research that examines the physiologic effects of meditation, therefore, is superfluous to this discussion. Scientific research that documents an accelerated evolution in the consciousness of meditators is minimal. These outcomes are not subject to quantitative analysis. However, there is extensive documentation of this phenomenon in the world literature—for example, in the chronicles of saints and mystics from all ages.

Prayer is a practice that differs substantively from meditation. It involves active supplication for a certain outcome. Again, it is not relevant to examine the existing research on the outcomes of prayer. From the evolutionary perspective, it would seem that prayer has less value for accelerating the evolution of consciousness than does meditation. Prayer is an active mental state, with the mind focused on a desired outcome. This state of mind may interfere with, rather than facilitate, openness to cosmic consciousness. However, the mind is a more subtle and powerful energy than the body. This is, no doubt, why intercessory prayer has been demonstrated scientifically to reduce morbidity and mortality in the context of a variety of health problems.[38]

CONCLUSION

True healing does not occur in an instant. It is the culmination of a long process of evolution that spans many lifetimes. Patience is a prerequisite to success, if one is attempting to accelerate the normal pace of development. One should not expect cure of disease. Healing is very different than curing. However, one can expect, as one becomes more in resonance with the highest consciousness, that greater inner and outer harmony and balance will unfold. Ultimately, this will lead to a state in which the presence or absence of disease is of little significance. Healing will occur regardless.

POSTSCRIPT

We have presented a perspective on life that encompasses the entire universe. Life is a school of evolution. Humans are units of conscious energy evolving, through all the experiences that they encounter, into greater knowledge, feeling, and power. Further, everything in the universe is an evolving unit of conscious energy. Through the experiences of health and illness, we find messages that help us in our evolutionary journey. We see our lack of inner and outer harmony and our lack of balance. The effort to learn the lessons brought by these experiences is an essential activity in the gradual but steady blossoming of the inner self. When we find our inner self, we realize that it is simply an aspect of a larger reality that supports the universe. Wisdom, and ultimately love, dawn. May we find peace and joy in the lessons brought by life!

REFERENCES

1. Aurobind, S. (1970). *The life divine*. Pondicherry, India: Sri Aurobindo Ashram Trust.
2. Ramananda, S. (1956). *Evolutionary spiritualism*. Bisalpur, India: Sadhana Karyalaya.
3. Ramananda, S. (1954). *Evolutionary outlook on life*. Bisalpur, India: Sadhana Karyalaya.
4. Ramananda, S. (n.d.). *Evolutionary sadhana*. Unpublished manuscript.
5. Teilhard de Chardin, P. (1970). *Activation of energy*. (R. Hague, Trans.) London: Collins.
6. Teilhard de Chardin, P. (1969). *Human energy*. (R. Hague, Trans.). New York: Harcourt Brace Jovanovich.
7. Teilhard de Chardin, P. (1965). *The phenomenon of man*. (B. Wall, Trans.). New York: Harper.
8. Kauffman, S. (1992). *The origins of order: Self-organization and selection in evolution*. New York: Oxford University Press.
9. Kauffman, S. (1996). *At home in the universe: The search for the laws of self-organization and complexity*. New York: Oxford University Press.
10. Sheldrake, R. (1981). *A new science of life: The hypothesis of morphic resonance*. Los Angeles: J. P. Tarcher.
11. Sheldrake, R. (1988). *The presence of the past: Morphic resonance and the habits of nature*. New York: Times Books.
12. Sheldrake, R. (1990). *The rebirth of nature: The greening of science and God*. London: Random Century Group.
13. Capra, F. (1975). *The tao of physics: An exploration of the parallels between modern physics and eastern mysticism*. Boulder: Shambala.
14. Capra, F. (1997). *The web of life: A new scientific understanding of living systems*. New York: Anchor Books.
15. Prigogine, I. (1980). *From being to becoming: Time and complexity in the physical sciences*. San Francisco: Freeman.
16. Denton, M. (1998). *Nature's destiny: How the laws of biology reveal purpose in nature*. New York: Simon and Schuster.
17. Davies, P. (1993). *The mind of God: The scientific basis for a rational world*. New York: Simon & Schuster Trade.

18. Murphy, M. (1993). *The future of the body: Explorations into the further evolution of human nature.* Los Angeles: J. P. Tarcher.

19. Rogers, M. (1970). *An introduction to the theoretical basis of nursing.* Philadelphia: F. A. Davis.

20. Rogers, M. (1987). Rogers' science of unitary human beings. In R. Parse (Ed.) *Nursing science: Major paradigms, theories, and critiques.* Philadelphia: Saunders.

21. Rogers, M. (1990). Nursing: Science of unitary, irreducible human beings: Update 1990. In E. A. M. Barrett (Ed.), *Visions of Rogers' science-based nursing.* New York: National League for Nursing.

22. Rogers, M. (1994). "Nursing science evolves." In M. Madrid & E.A.M. Barrett (Eds.), *Rogers' scientific art of nursing practice.* New York: National League for Nursing.

23. Bohm, D. (1995). *The undivided universe.* London: Routledge & Kegan Paul.

24. Bohm, D. (1996). *Wholeness and the implicate order.* London: Routledge & Kegan Paul.

25. Waldrop, M. M. (1992). *Complexity: The emerging science at the edge of order and chaos.* New York: Simon & Schuster.

26. Morse, M. (1991). *Closer to the light: Learning from near death experiences of children.* New York: Random House.

27. Moody, R. A. (1976). *Life after life.* New York: Bantam Doubleday Dell.

28. Gebser, J. (1986). *The ever-present origin.* (N. Barstad & A. Mickunas, Trans.). Athens, OH: Ohio University Press.

29. Dossey, L. (2000). Distant nonlocal awareness: A different kind of DNA. *Alternative Therapies in Health and Medicine* 6(6): 10–14, 102–110.

30. Gould, S. J. (1992). *Ever since Darwin: Reflections in natural history.* New York: Norton.

31. Einstein, A. (1949). *The world as I see it.* (A. Harris, Trans.). New York: Philosophical Library.

32. Eddington, A. (1929). *Science and the unseen world.* New York: MacMillan.

33. Schrodinger, E. (1956). *What is life? And other scientific essays.* Garden City, NY: Doubleday.

34. Jeans, J. H. (1958). *Physics and philosophy.* Ann Arbor, MI: Univ. of Michigan Press.

35. Stevenson, I. (1974). *Twenty cases suggestive of reincarnation.* (2nd ed.). Charlottesville, VA: University Press of Virginia.

36. Pizzorno, J. and Murray, M. (1992). *Textbook of natural medicine.* Seattle: Bastyr University Press.

37. Johnston-Taylor, E., and M. Amenta, (1994). Preliminary results of hospice nurse spiritual care survey. *Fanfare* 8(3),9.

38. Byrd, R. C. (1997). Positive therapeutic effects of intercessory prayer in a coronary care unit population, *Alternative Therapies in Health and Medicine* 3(6), 87–90.

39. Kubler-Ross, E. (1969). *On death and dying.* New York: Macmillan.

40. Watts, A. (1961). *Psychotherapy east and west.* New York: Ballantine Books.

41. James, W. (1958). *The varieties of religious experience.* New York: The New American Library.

42. Richardson, M. A. et. al. (1997). Coping, life attitudes, and immune responses to imagery and group support after breast cancer. *Alternative Therapies in Health and Medicine* 3(5), 62–70.

43. Mackenzie, E. R. et. al. (2000). Spiritual support and psychological well-being: Older adults' perceptions of the religion and health connection. *Alternative Therapies in Health and Medicine* 6(6), 37–45.

44. Nightingale, F. (1860/1969). *Notes on nursing: What it is and what it is not.* New York: Dover.

45. Spinoza, B. (1949). *Ethics.* New York: Hafner.

46. Prem, S. K. (1969). *The yoga of the Bhagavat Gita.* London: Stuart & Watkins.

47. Jowett, S. (trans. (1892). *Dialogues of Plato, vol I— Phaedrus.* (3rd ed.). Oxford: Oxford University Press.

48. Moody, R. A. (1976). *Life after life: The investigation of a phenomenon—survival of bodily death.* New York: Bantam Books.

49. Moody, R. A. (1977). *Reflections on life after life.* Atlanta: Mockingbird Books.

50. Osis, K. & E. Haraldsson. (1977). *At the hour of death.* New York: Avon Books.

51. Fenwick, P. (1997). *The truth in the light.* New York: Berkely Books.

52. Evans-Wentz, W. Y. (Ed.). (1957). *The Tibetan book of the dead.* New York: Oxford University Press.

53. Borman, W. (1990). *The other side of death: Upanishadic eschatology.* Delhi, India: Indian Books Center.

54. Schroeder-Sheku, T. (2001). Music thanatology and spiritual care for the dying—interview. *Alternative Therapies in Health and Medicine* 7(1), 68–77.

55. Sarno, J. E. (1991). *Healing back pain.* New York: Warner Books.

56. Freeman, L. W. & G. F. Lawlis (2001). Exercise as an alternative therapy. In L. W. Freeman & G. F. Lawlis, *Mosby's guide to complementary and alternative medicine: A research-based approach.* St. Louis: Mosby.

57. Freeman, L. (2001). Massage therapy. In L. W. Freeman & G. F. Lawlis, *Mosby's guide to complementary and alternative medicine: A research-based approach.* St. Louis: Mosby.

58. Hahnemann, S. (1982/1810). *Organon of medicine.* (J. Kunzli et. al., Trans.). Los Angeles: J. P. Tarcher.

59. Jacobs, J. et. al. (1994). Treatment of acute childhood diarrhea with homeopathic medicine: A randomized clinical trial in Nicaragua. *Pediatrics* 93, 719.

60. Reilly, D., et. al. (1994). Is evidence for homeopathy reproducible? *Lancet* 344, 1601.

61. Lu, H. C. (Trans.) (1978). *The yellow emperor's classic of internal medicine and the difficult classic.* Vancouver: Academy of Oriental Heritage.

62. Freeman, L. W. (2001). Acupuncture. In L. W. Freeman & G. F. Lawlis, *Mosby's guide to complementary and alternative medicine: A research-based approach.* St. Louis: Mosby.

63. Lad, V. (1986). *Ayurveda: The science of self-healing.* Santa Fe: Lotus Press.

64. Freeman, L. W. (2001). Therapeutic touch. In L. W. Freeman & G. F. Lawlis, *Mosby's guide to complementary and alternative medicine: A research-based approach.* St. Louis: Mosby.

65. Quinn, J. F. (1984). Therapeutic touch as energy exchange: Testing the theory. *Advances in Nursing Science* 6, 42.

66. Samarel, N., et. al. (1998). Effects of dialogue and therapeutic touch on preoperative and postoperative experiences of breast cancer surgery: An exploratory study, *Oncology Nursing Forum* 28(8),1369.

67. Wirth, D. P. (1992). The effect of non-contact therapeutic touch on the healing rate of full thickness dermal wounds. *Subtle Energies* 1(1), 1.

68. Turner, J. G., et. al. (1998). The effect of therapeutic touch on pain and anxiety in burn patients. *Journal of Advanced Nursing* 28(1), 10.

69. Graham, H. *Complementary therapies in context: The psychology of healing.* (1999). London: Jessica Kingsley.

70. Burns, S. J., et. al. (2001). A pilot study into the therapeutic effects of music therapy at a cancer help center. *Alternative Therapies in Health and Medicine* 7(1), 48–56.

INDEX

DATE DUE

OCT 1 9 2010		
OCT 1 9 2010		
NOV 1 1 2010		

HIGHSMITH 45231